THE AQUARIAN
ROSARY

Other books by Carol E. Parrish-Harra:

The New Age Handbook on Death and Dying
Rev. Parrish-Harra offers insights from her ministries with terminally ill patients and their families,
as well as her own near-death experience.

Messengers of Hope
After being identified as a "walk-in" by Ruth Mont-
gomery in *Threshold to Tomorrow*, Carol reveals her
mission to create a spiritual community.

**The Book of Rituals—Personal and
Planetary Transformation**
This highly original work presents rituals involving
prayer, song, chanting, dance, and meditation for
each full moon period and for major festivals.

The New Dictionary of Spiritual Thought
This valuable reference work contains more than
1,100 of the world's most important Western and
Eastern esoteric and spiritual definitions.

The AQUARIAN ROSARY

Reviving The Art of Mantra Yoga

Rev. Carol E. Parrish-Harra, Ph.D.

SPARROW HAWK PRESS

Tahlequah, Oklahoma

Sparrow Hawk Press
11 Summit Ridge Drive, Tahlequah, OK 74464

Book design and cover: Dianna K. Christenson
Illustrations: Cedar Carrier

Library of Congress Catalog Card Number 87-063437
ISBN 0-945027-01-X

Dedicated to

THE MOTHER OF THE WORLD
May we grow in an understanding of
the Divine Feminine Principle

Table Of Contents

Illustrations

FOREWORD

I was raised Lutheran. We ate meat on Fridays and prided ourselves in not being Catholic. As a teenager I dated a Catholic girl who always carried a rosary. I thought it was just so much mumbo-jumbo. We argued about it. Little did I know that years later I would be saying a Rosary for peace and justice regularly with a group of Protestants every Wednesday night at midnight and finding it a very meaningful experience. Much of the content of the rosary we use is quite different from the one my girlfriend had, but it is better suited for our religious sensitivities and spiritual needs.

There are many versions of the rosary. Usually these are designed for the same people to use under differing circumstances. What humanity needs at this time are many different rosaries, each one worded appropriately for different groups of people so that more and more of God's people can experience the benefits of this special form of prayer. It was with this thought in mind that I greeted *The Aquarian Rosary* by Carol W. Parrish-Harra with joyful gratitude. It will surely find a ready group of users who would perhaps never otherwise get involved saying the rosary in its more traditional forms.

Humanity has reached the point in its development when it has become of vital importance that the masculine and the feminine be blended and balanced. It was necessary for a time, in the Divine Plan, that the masculine be allowed to develop lop-sidedly so that it might take a firm hold in the personality.

In this way it would not be lost and swallowed up in the feminine—which in its archetypal form is awesome. This development would, however, if continued, become evermore destructive in its one-sidedness. Now the blending can be accomplished without the feminine being completely overwhelming. Response to the influence of Mary will bring out the positive feminine attributes in people, and saying the rosary is one way in which She can work Her vibratory influence in us.

Master Jesus, the Christ, has called us to be members of one united body—the "invisible church." We are to join in spirit with all the saints in heaven and all the just on earth who in all times and places have praised the Holy Name. In saying the rosary the Spirit of God helps us in praising the Holy Mother worthily that, in devotion to the ideal symbolized in the Immaculate Heart of Mary, we may find that which is the hope of God's becoming individualized as we thereby become manifestations of God's love.

As we try to keep abreast of world news, get ourselves informed regarding the true state of world conditions and the plight of people everywhere and indeed the plight of the planet itself, and as we try to be alert to the signs of the times, we are admonished by the "Lady from Heaven," who has been appearing in apparitions around the world with greater and greater frequency as to express a sense of urgency, to say the rosary frequently—every day if possible.

We are reminded in the prayer of St. Bernard, which is often included as The Memorare in the rosary, that never was it known that anyone who flees to the protection of the most compassionate Virgin Mother, implores Her help or seeks Her intercession is left unaided.

Saying the rosary regularly, like all disciplined prayer, requires heartfelt dedication. Some individuals get discouraged and stop coming because they do not see the results. We have been told, however, by those from realms above, that it is possible to prevent much suffering in the world as it goes through its painful transition or birthing process if even a handful of people are filled with love and sincere dedication.

I was struck by the many statements in the first four chapters which seem truly inspired. They will have a preparing effect in the soul. I suggest that you read these chapters carefully three times at spaced intervals.

Another treat awaits the reader of *The Aquarian Rosary* in chapter eight. I have long enjoyed Corinne Heline's works and was glad to see that her writings on the rosary were included in their entirety.

The part bringing most definite and lasting effects is the actual gathering together as a group to say the rosary, which in this case is one of fifteen decades (or could be used as three separate five-decade rosaries on different occasions). It is found in chapters five, six and seven of The Technique section which could be excerpted for handy use.

Your task, reader, if you feel drawn to the form and content of *The Aquarian Rosary*, is to find a like-minded group that you can join in saying the rosary regularly. If you can't find such a group in your area, then the call to you is clear: **form one!**

James Ulness, Ph.D.

Acknowledgements

The author wishes to give special thanks to those who worked with such dedication to gather this material. I thank Richard and Dianna Kay for their hours at the computer, and Cedar for her lovely, feminine illustrations. My gratitude to Grace and Nita for their reading and commenting; and to Mary Beth, who arrived just in time to add necessary expertise to the efforts in process. To the persons at the Village who say the rosary, share their experience and support the emerging feminine in themselves, you are part of my heart and part of this book.

Preface

The planet entered a period of change on August 17, 1987, and will rapidly increase its struggle to adjust to a new frequency. We are being caught up in a heightened awareness by the cosmic influence whether we are ready or not.

From August 17, 1987, until December 21, 2012, we shall pass through a period of transition, a cleansing. We, as a body of cellular life, have to be able to live together as interlocking cells at the human level. All life on the planet has to participate in the experience of preserving the planetary body. It is the role of humankind to act as the intelligence of the planet—the brain cells through which the Higher Mind can act.

Humanity is being guided to seek and utilize invocations, rituals and a mental comprehension that will guide it in this adjustment. We are told repeatedly that the incoming energy will disrupt, incite lower or hidden, repressed emotions and contribute to mental illness, crime and disease. Rituals of great love and spiritual power which can be easily used with large numbers of people are not only needed to help them touch into the spiritual forces of Will, Love-Wisdom and Active Intelligence, but will prove to be stabilizing tools of transformation during this critical quarter century.

With these thoughts in mind, I offer the Aquarian Rosary as one tool to aid humanity in the Great Work that confronts it.

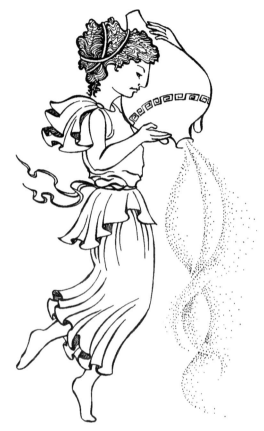

Symbol of the Aquarian Waterbearer

The Era of the Cosmic Mother is the time of a great Age of Enlightenment. The Star of Her Light will flash forth to awaken the Christ hidden within the Children of Humanity. Hear Her call. Arise and shine. Rejoice!

Part I

INTRODUCTION

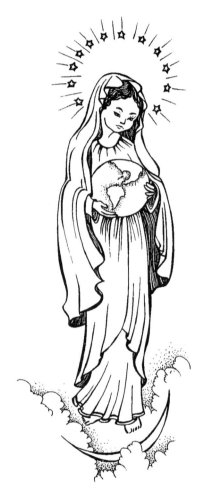

The Christian Virgin Mary
nurtures humanity

Chapter 1

The Little-Known Importance of the Rosary

Many spiritual teachers are currently receiving impressions for aspirants of various paths to turn to the rosary as a modern chant, a tool for invoking spiritual grace. One might think of this use of grace as spiritual power. The concept of grace has been largely related to freeing from bondage or limitation.

Healing is a powerful form of grace that uses the outpouring of holy force to break through unfinished business and re-establish a more desired, more liberated state. Perhaps we can see a relationship between humanity's need for healing and assistance at this time and the invocation of grace through this familiar series of prayers. The prayers used are not just memorized words; they are positive, beneficial rote and repetitive expressions used to still the basic self while the mental nature pierces the veil into the high consciousness, in contemplation of the pearls of wisdom contained in the rosary's teaching parables.

Since the majority of people of the past could not read or count, beads became the most accurate way to record prayer repetitions. Beads serve to keep the physical aspect participating while the attention is gradually lifted into higher realms. While the fingers move on the beads, the heart focuses on devotion and the mind contemplates the parables and the quality of the spiritual life they suggest. By invocation, the power of the higher planes is invited into our lives collectively and individually to do a holy work. Each system or spiritual tradition has its beads. The East, even today, uses the *mala*. The Hebrew tradition has its *phylactery* which invokes physical action, repetitive prayer and the holding of thoughts in contemplation/meditation. The Huna had the *worry stone* to be fingered.

The Western rosary was introduced in 13th century Europe and provided one of the first introductions to seed thought meditation within the Christian tradition. Originally called a *rosarium*, it consisted of four different forms until the first synthesis occurred in the 14th century.

Henry de Kalhes, a Carthusian monk, organized it into Our Fathers and 150 Hail Marys, with one Our Father between each decade of Hail Marys (Latin). In 1409 Saint Dominic (the Prussian) brought the rosary into more common practice and added a thought from the life of Jesus or Mary to each of the Hail Marys. By the end of the century the use of this rosary had spread throughout Europe.

While many variations have been enjoyed, the manner of saying the rosary has changed little since the Middle Ages. An awareness of the energy work increases as the chant builds, developing into a rhythm-building style that is not clearly spoken in words but establishes a smooth, rapid cadence. It has been repeatedly stated that the rosary is a sacred ritual whereby all of God's children can find their way back to their immaculate conception in the heart of the Cosmic Virgin. This statement in itself is a grand seed thought.

Wisdom teachings tell us that the physical, emotional and mental aspects of a human being must be integrated for spiritualization to occur. As our nature experiences this effort of focus, another work is going on out of sight. The personality is being prepared for the experience of new awareness.

The Rosary and Mantra Yoga

A *mantra* is a program of incantations spoken to the subconscious to reprogram and train one for new awareness. Mantra Yoga is the practice of using mantras, affirmations, prayers or chants as a technique to create union (yoga) between levels of self: spirit and matter, or lesser self and high self. Jesus used the word *yoke* in the Bible to signify the same concept, speaking as a teacher of the yoga He had to offer. He said, "Take my yoke upon you and learn of me...for my yoke is easy and my burden is light."[1]

Yoga is commonly thought of as a physical practice, but it is not. An older form of yoga called *Hatha* Yoga does use physical postures (or asanas), but the contemporary practice of yoga focuses on the mind and emotions, rather than the physical body.

How can repeating mantras, prayers and words of power or holy names be of help to us? Remember that everything is vibration. The higher the vibration to which we are responding, the higher and holier a space we are in. Aspirants in the Eastern traditions from earliest times have been taught to keep the name of God on their lips. The chanting of the names of holy ones is designed to uplift our vibration and attune us to the saint or sage of our devotion. There is a wonderful story that when Mahatma Gandhi was assassinated, as he was struck and fell dead, he muttered, "Ram," the deity to whom he was devoted. What a blessing!

---

1 Matt. 11:28-30, AV

Sound (or vibration) is the most powerful force in the world. The scriptures tell us, "In the beginning was the Word, and the Word was with God, and the Word was God."[1] Ancient peoples utilized sound and tones for many purposes; the science of vibration is just beginning to be understood by modern scientists.

The derivation of words holds such esoteric importance that Kabalists of old studied words hidden within words to find concealed meanings. We can analyze the word *spiritual* in this way. *Spirit* comes from the Latin word meaning breath; *ritual*, also Latin in origin, means rites. The combination spirit-ritual means breath-rites. It is interesting that we often refer to the Holy Spirit as the Holy Breath; *The Aquarian Gospel of Jesus the Christ*[2] always uses this term. The word *spiritual*, then, implies the need for rituals to increase the Breath or Spirit within us. Chanting is one such ritual.

The reason for chanting is to spiritualize the consciousness through invocation of higher energies. Chanting does a little-understood work on both our emotions and the lower levels of mind. There is a sensitive, powerful body of energy in the emotional level that stirs easily; this is called the *astral body*. When its energy is pure and positive, it elevates, moving us from emotion to devotion, then toward aspiration.

---

1 John 1:1, RSV
2 Levi, Marina del Ray, Calif.: DeVorss & Co., 1907

When we are filled with pain, it stirs and seeks to find relief, to facilitate cleansing or healing.

As we chant in simple, repetitive ways while encouraging emotional-devotional energy and thoughts, we touch into this reservoir of spiritual power to actualize a linkage to deeper levels of awareness. This connects us to the human group mind or collective unconscious, that unaware part of us that is one with the Source. The experience stirs and cleanses us emotionally and, through the use of *seed thoughts*, allows us to penetrate the Divine Intelligence. Thus we grow and become the very virtues we hold in our minds.

Entering an atmosphere which has been prepared by such a spiritual technique has a healthful effect on participants, and change occurs to the degree that one's emotions are moved by the experience. If we actively participate, we are inviting its influence to become more real for us. If we choose not to participate, we will still receive a share of the *lift* through the environment's action upon us. We each benefit only to the degree we permit; this is an important key to experiencing any ritual.

The rosary is a ritualistic tool of transition and invocation. Use it in this way. When in doubt, fill yourself with its positive force called spiritual power.

Transformation, Transmutation, Transfiguration

Spiritual teachings repeatedly refer to transformation, transmutation and transfiguration. While closely related, the terms are not the same; each pertains to a different process.

The first work is the *transformation* of the personality so that it aligns with a pattern appropriate to spiritual life. Think of this as sensitizing the person so the incoming spiritual forces can have impact. This is the level which modern churches try to influence. The esoteric Christian tradition, however, concerns itself with the inner work of birthing the Christ-Within, rather than the path of dogma and particular denominational positions. *Esoteric* means an *inner* or *out-of-sight* process. Esoteric Christians believe that Christianity as offered to humanity by Master Jesus is a transformational process to enlightenment; the teachings and practices should lead us to the transpersonal level of consciousness. This is the Divine-Within which brings us to "the mind that is in Christ Jesus be also in each of us,"[1] so that ultimately we may each be able to say, "I and my Father are one."[2]

While most Christians focus on the outer or exoteric tradition, the time will come in their growth and individualization when they will

1 A paraphrase of Phil. 2:5, (KJV): "Let this mind be in you, which was also in Christ Jesus"
2 John 10:30, AV

demand more of their religious practice than words and songs. They will want to penetrate into the holy space where transformation can occur. Chanting the rosary produces a vibrational change that allows the inner processes to cleanse and clear and energizes the changes that may occur. This is just a part of a larger lifestyle for the serious spiritual student, but it is an empowering part. Here one leaves the *religious* realm and begins to deal with *spiritual* practices. The religious gives us keys and guides the outer life by dogma; the essence of self will ultimately seek food for its own hunger.

Meditation is a powerful tool to increase sensitivity to higher vibrations. Energizing the personality with high and holy words of power increases the response to higher influences. The light evoked stimulates the light of the cells, or dense body; and the light of spirit and the matter of physical life move toward balance. The effects are ones of healing, increased sensitivity, development of astral senses and flashes of intuition—a certain radiance develops.

This invocation of spiritual energy also clears and cleanses the astral and mental vehicles. As the astral reflects the feelings and the mind focuses upward, their refined frequencies capture and reflect the higher. Devotion fills the astral vehicle with love and energies of the soul, and negative emotions are released or neutralized. Love fills the life as higher aspirations begin to guide. As light penetrates the mental vehicles, illusions that obscure clear-seeing and the wisdom of the higher plan dissolve. The mind more faithfully reflects the high self level of awareness, facilitating the cleansing work; heart, mind and body begin to harmonize. The aspirant keeps self charged with Light, Love and Spiritual Power for the purpose of transforming the physical life.

Transmutation is the process of reworking the physical, emotional and mental levels of personality through changes in the very substance of the vehicles. As the cleansing of each level takes place, there is an actual transmutation from *matter* to *light*. The body, now much more reflective of heart and mind, gradually becomes a delicate receiver set for high frequencies. The refined emotional nature becomes a reflective source of energy that responds enthusiastically to flashes of light from the higher. As the holy names and words of spiritual power are spoken in a contemplative, devotional, quiet and sincere manner, both *matter* and *consciousness* vibrate to a higher frequency. The instrument adjusts or adapts to handle the frequencies the individual is evoking. In other words, the etheric counterpart of the physical vehicle becomes clearer and has more impact on the physical receiver set. The aura around the person increases in its glow or vibrancy.

H. P. Blavatsky said, "Manas is spiritual self-consciousness." This high consciousness cannot express itself in the lower world without a reflective device. It is our human mind, or *lower manas*, which serves as that device. It is therefore the task of the lower manas, the thinking personality, to dissipate and paralyze the properties of the material form which hinder the light. It is the *kama-manas*, the lower ego, that would be deluded into the false belief of independent existence.

As the illusion of human intelligence lessens, the mind that is in Christ Jesus evolves. This is the mind that *thinketh in the heart*, also spoken of as *the heart behind the heart*. Feeling (heart) and knowing (mind) blend, transmuting the receiving vehicles and imbuing them with harmonious abilities dedicated to service. The abilities of the spiritual ones are disclosed. "Greater things than these shall ye do" becomes a real potential, rather than wishful thinking. This mind, attuned to Divine Mind, is a result of the transmuting process.

Extended consciousness builds the thread connecting the higher manas with the kama-manas, producing a spirit-filled consciousness living within matter. The power of the human ego is to cleanse the personality of confusion, distortion and error (sin) if it so chooses. It becomes a real effort for the sincere disciple to do this cleansing for the self; and it is a great work for awakened ones on behalf of the many in a time when there is so much to do—and so few to do it.

As invocation continues, the **transfiguration** from human to divine follows. The new Adam, or God-man, is born.

The Three-brain Concept

For those who have been exposed to the three-brain concept of human evolution, I offer another link. It has been postulated that the animal part of our being operates from the **reptilian brain**. This is the level of intelligence that is responsible for the sympathetic nervous system, which keeps us involuntarily breathing, digesting food and performing other automatic functions. In order to develop, this brain requires repetition and formality. Its greatest concern is survival.

The second brain in human development is the mammalian, or **mid-brain**. It works not only on a one-to-one basis but more specifically with group relationships. It knows the need for socialization and is aware that the biological system links us to the species and all of life. Here the powerful and easily aroused emotional sense helps us relate to the group. In addition to repetition and formality, the mid-brain needs movement to feel its rich connection to the Oneness. The use of rote movement helps strengthen the mid-brain to better relate one to another. This is the seat of self-esteem.

Joseph Chilton Pearce, author of *Magical Child*, *The Crack in the Cosmic Egg* and *Bond of Power*, suggests that the mid-brain has been weakened in childhood by the neglect of emotional development and premature pursuit of the intellectual. This has resulted in the loss of our "realization of right relationship to one another and the whole." He suggests that if we are misprogrammed we will always misfunction. The mid-brain contains the fault.

The breakdown we see in society today is the outgrowth of underdevelopment and misprogramming of the mid-brain. All our connections at a social level seem to depend on this sense of group appreciation. The ancients knew that children have an innate sense of their group and used the patterns of child development as a guide for spiritual development. In the beginning the aspirant was required to fill the life with simple, repetitive activities. To those with other interests, the aspirant's life seemed reduced to simplicity and monotony. As this base was developed, one was guided to understand his relationship with all of life, particularly to his group brothers.[1] Sacred texts are filled with specific references to our all being parts of one body and the concepts of love one another and the golden rule. Conceptualizing God as Father-Mother of all humanity fosters this idea.

---

1 "Group brothers" is used in esoteric terminology to denote those with whom we find ourselves specifically linked in our spiritual growth. It is not sexist—it is used by male and female, convents and monasteries, somewhat like a "Class of 1987" or a number evolving together. The human and angelic kingdoms are brothers, as in "Am I my brother's keeper?"

The third and newest portion of the human brain is the **neocortex**, the center of ego structure since human individualization. It is divided into left and right hemispheres: the right hemisphere is imaginative, intuitive, gentle and feminine, while the left hemisphere is rational, cognitive, analytical and masculine in nature. Due to individual life experiences, we are usually more in touch with one hemisphere than the other. Most of us are products of an intellectual society and a system that rewards abilities of the masculine hemisphere. We are prepared to believe only what we can validate, operating within a code of masculinity. As we experience flashes that connect us to the right hemisphere, it is easy for the left hemisphere to convince us that our imaginations have gone awry. This can happen during moments of great love, positive emotion and intuitive insight or in the spiritual context of visions, perceptions of God and the soul or the sensing of a part of God's great Plan in some way.

As we evolve into more intelligent and creative beings, the two hemispheres begin to *arc*. Those who have made this mental connection are highly resourceful, exceptionally intelligent and capable. The active use of resources from both hemispheres allows us to evolve into the wonderful beings we are intended to be.

It is the third brain that opens for inspiration as the other levels are prepared, cleansed and made whole. Here we must clear the unreal to find the real. We have to know and understand. We have to "let go and let God" in our inner lives. We must be excited about our inner life for it to reveal itself. It is creative and dynamic, but expansion of consciousness does not happen to the lukewarm person. A fervent desire from the heart and the emotional level is necessary to excite the mental. The rosary can be a useful tool to fan the flame of the human heart so that devotion may rise like a sweet smoke before the Cosmic Heart, energizing emerging patterns of life for a more fully-aware humanity. The poised mind, made single-minded in its search, pierces the veil; and the chalice (receptive mind) catches the flash. The masculine left hemisphere is focused and the feminine right hemisphere is receptive. As the droplet of divine realization comes, it can happen. *All is ready, Master. Come.*

The rosary is a way of using seed thoughts within an environment of spiritual vibration and aspiration to help us pull the left and right hemispheres together. Then we can experience that arc of light that flashes from the higher manas. Our brain desires new and creative materials. Seed thoughts are designed to put us in a posture to receive guidance from higher levels. Breakthroughs can occur which provide solutions, creative insights, ideas for inventions and guidance for individuals. This keeps the mental mechanism of the species developing; it is the place of *straight knowledge* or revelation.

Chanting with beads or physical movement is the simplest available exercise to bring about such results for humanity. It is a discipline that becomes an adventure as one learns to sense the non-physical shift or change. If one cannot wait one hour for the Lord, then one is not a leader of the race. If we have such ready tools, can we take them up and do such a service? Hopefully the Divine Feminine, which is manifesting so frequently as the Mother Presence in many parts of the world at this time, will find us ready.

The mantra is a program spoken to the subconscious, opening the gateway so we can rescript and enjoy the transcendent state of mind. We are opening to the God Imminent to fill, repair and replenish us. Repeating mantras correctly causes hemispheric balance. Insights, realizations, healing and inner knowing are the result.

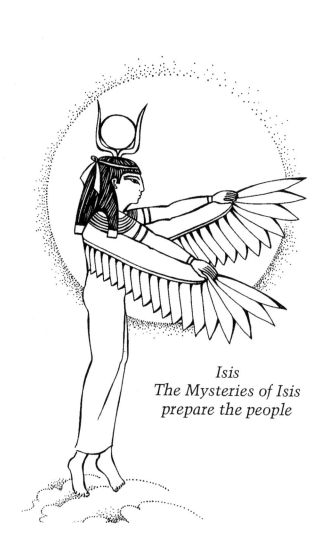

Isis
The Mysteries of Isis
prepare the people

Chapter 2

The Divine Feminine

Before the era which the Bible calls the Age of the Patriarchs and stretching back into earlier dim recesses of time, the Great Mother ruled humanity and nurtured Her people. To these early ancestors the female simply was the source of life. Only a woman could bring forth children and the mother's milk that provided *life* for the newly born.

In ancient times the goddess with her boundless mystery of life was considered the creator, the lawgiver, the wise counselor, the bounty of Mother Earth, the dark womb to which humanity returned after death, the Queen of Heaven, All. Within this mysterious life-figure all opposites were embraced, loved and understood.

Both the productive aspect of nature and the growing, developing aspect could be accepted.

Today so much mental rationale has been developed that we must now stimulate an equal amount of love-compassion to offset the coldness. The traits of excessive masculinity have moved into negative over-expression: competition without compassion, brute force, power without temperance, war without mercy or nobility and lack of respect and appreciation for emotion, nature and the life of the earth are all part of the absence of love for the Divine Feminine Principle. We must bring in the love that is needed in order to "thinketh in the heart."

A profound change in human consciousness must emerge upon our planet. As the Aquarian Age makes its presence felt and life itself is threatened, humanity must call out to the Divine Mother for help—to grant us peace. Having come to the brink of destruction, humanity must turn its eyes toward the Great Cosmic Mother for protection and preservation. A simple awareness becomes increasingly clear that we need the wisdom of this feminine principle to help us bring to consciousness the refined, loving and nurturing part of our selves to save ourselves from ourselves. The first step will be to place emphasis on the heart and that feminine force it represents.

It is the work of awakened ones to use the tools readily available to prevent continued damage to the human psyche and eliminate the danger-

ous use of mind without heart. The Aquarian
Rosary can be a powerful prayer formula to build
a greater subconscious awareness of our relationship to the Cosmic Mother. This will spiritualize or tenderize the behavior of the force
that has been set into motion. In performing the
ritual of the rosary, we are consciously seeking
to heal our separation from the Divine Feminine
that nurtures and protects. We are strengthening
the relationship between humanity, nature, the
planet and the Mother principle; and we are invoking from the great wholeness a positive
memory of humanity in right-relationship to the
All.

The ritual of invoking the Divine Feminine is a
work of service for all of humanity, not only for
oneself. Each person doing such work achieves
in two ways: first, his or her own personality is
filled with the energy evoked, which affects the
nature through incoming power and grace; second, the energy of the Divine Feminine is also
drawn into the human group mind.

Contemplation of the rosary as a spiritual technique increases our understanding of the benefits that accrue to humanity as it regains respect
for the feminine principle. We find a reservoir of
healing, comfort, tenderness, sensitivity and
protection. We strengthen our appreciation of
feminine dignity and purity and begin to re-establish worthy, spiritual role-models to em-
power the woman of the new age. We turn to the

feminine strengths and invoke a return to
balance and wholeness.

The Babaji that Paramahansa Yogananda talks of
in his *Autobiography of a Yogi*[1] spoke regularly
of the Divine Feminine influence as Divine
Mother. While embodied in Haidakhan, India,
Babaji emphasized the need for us to turn our
hearts to the Divine Mother in the form of
Shakti. Receive Shakti from the Divine Mother
and this grace will be protective of those attuned
to her. Having been deeply touched by this mod-
ern-day saint, I add the power of his influence to
our study of the rosary.

The following comments are published in *Our
Lady of Fatima Revelation: Divine Mother
Speaks:*[2]

> If you want salvation, the Virgin Mary says
> pray on the rosary (call this "japa," if you
> wish) and seek the Grace and Indulgence of
> the Universal Mother through penance.

> In many speeches and in personal advice,
> Shri Babaji said the only salvation during
> this Mahakranti/Revolution is japa (simi-
> lar to reciting the rosary) and absolute
> devotion to the Supreme Mother (Shakti).

> It is therefore very clear that with things
> around the world reflecting a crazy mani-
> festation of sin and ignorance, Shri Babaji

---

1 Los Angeles: Self-Realization Fellowship, 1946
2 As translated from Italian by Tuka Ram, Haidakhan,
   India, date unknown

said the same things as those stated by the
Holy Mother at Fatima. It is uncanny (or divine???) that three sources (Nostradamus,
Haidakhan Babaji and Our Lady of Fatima)
should make such similar predictions at
different times and in different places.

Beware! Be alert!... Do japa; or say the rosary! And by Shri Babaji's Grace we will
withstand any evil and demonic forces
with poise, courage and spiritual strength.

Marvelous in its inception and stupendous
in its awful aspects, the Mahakranti/Revo-
lution is a great lesson: do NOT forget to
pray to the Divine Mother (Shakti) and con-
centrate on japa, and your salvation will be
assured.

In her book, *Kundalini and the Third Eye*,[1] Ear-
lyne Chaney of the Astara School says, "The
traditional rosary chant is a prayer to the Blessed
Virgin Mary, who represents the feminine aspect
of God overshadowing the human lifewave of
souls evolving on this particular planet."

Peter Roche de Coppens in *The Nature and Use
of Ritual for Spiritual Attainment*[2] says of the
Hail Mary,

Short and simple as it is, (it) is one of
the...most important spiritual documents
containing profound esoteric knowledge
and a series of integrated and practical ex-
ercises designed to establish a break-

1 Upland, Calif.: Astara, 1980
2 St. Paul, Minn.: Llewellyn Publications, 1986

> through between the conscious and the su-
> perconscious, to fill the human aura with
> spiritual Light, and to harmonize man's
> human self with his Spiritual Self.
>
> Mary, therefore, represents the ideal
> woman, the perfection of the female prin-
> ciple, and the incarnation of the eternal
> feminine aspect—a part which we all have
> within our being.

The prolific writer-teacher, Corinne Heline, wrote such an important chapter on "The Mystic Rosary" that it has been reproduced in its entirety within this volume. She states, "The Blessed Virgin Mary belongs to no one church or creed, race or nation." The many apparitions, visitations and manifestations connected with the Virgin that are happening all over the planet today certainly bear witness to this statement. It is timely for us as the people of an awakening new era to call forth the feminine influence into our masculine-dominated awareness to promote wholeness and balance for humanity and our planet.

Pope John Paul declared 1987 a Marian Year for Peace. This means the year has been offered to Mary by the Pope, seeking her intercession on behalf of humanity. Interesting events are occurring around the world that are attracting our attention to Mary, the World Mother, as known to the Christian people.

June of 1987 marked the sixth anniversary of Mary's daily apparitions to the visionaries at

Medjugorje, Yugoslavia, which began June 24, 1981. Within the messages of these appearances Mary has beseeched humanity to respond to her through prayers, fasting, reconciliation with others, penance and the living of a spiritual lifestyle, as well as seeking growth within one's faith.

In the first three years of appearances in this remote part of Europe a million and a half persons came to worship—now it is that number in a year. Fr. Al Winshman (a priest of the Medjugorje Center, Loyola Retreat House, Faulkner, MD 20632) dedicated himself to making the messages of Mary known in the United States. While he was in Medjugorje he received this message to bring to the public:

> Dear children, Today also I am inviting you to prayer. You know, dear children, that God is granting special graces in prayer. Therefore, seek and pray, in order that you may be able to understand all I am giving you in this place. I am calling you to pray with your heart. You know, dear children, that without prayer you cannot comprehend all that God is planning through each one of you. And so pray! I want that through every one of you God's plan may be fulfilled, that all that God has given you in your hearts may increase. Therefore, pray that God's blessing may protect everyone of you from all the evil that is threatening you. I am blessing you, dear children. Thank you for your response to my call!

Another current event interested me to the degree that I went to Chicago to experience the phenomenon. In December, 1986, moisture appeared in the eyes and began streaming down the face of an icon in the St. Nicholas Albanian Orthodox Church, 2701 N. Narragansett Avenue. Painted in 1962 on canvas which was adhered to half-inch plywood, the icon radiates the presence of Love—Divine Feminine. In April of 1987 I experienced the energy of this one. The hushed vibrations of the room drew the devotees inward. Pure and radiant she made herself felt. As I stood watching the "tears" well in the eyes of the Madonna, I felt the warmth of my own tears. An usher told me there are about 400 manifestations occurring around the world involving Our Lady.

The tears have since ceased as a daily experience, but changes in the parish continue. The people register the touch. Money was not solicited, but donations came. Church officials set up a fund to be held in trust, with the interest going to soup kitchens in the city as a way to continue to nourish Her needy.

The Aquarian Age, the era of woman, returns respect to the feminine nature of humanity to unite the segregated aspects of life with what is needed to repair right-relationships: people to people, country to country, kingdom to kingdom. The worlds of nature and the populace of the planet must realize they are all Mother Earth's children. The Great Mother principle can be healing and tender but can also punish. The Earth will unloose destruction in order to cleanse itself; the children will become obedient to the laws of life. Through such a challenge, we mature to become law-abiding co-workers with that which produces life and protects us all.

The Cosmic Mother is working on the purple transmuting vibration to heal the subconscious of humanity in order to produce divine beings who will unite the planet and make it receptive to the Plan. She waits patiently for the awakened to turn their faces to the Light. The feminine principle is not to replace the masculine principle but is to be restored to value in itself. The age of enlightenment long promised will release honor and restore full dignity and power to the great stream of Life that manifests on our planet.

As we turn our hearts and minds toward the restoration of the Mother principle of the cosmos, we strengthen the connection between the cosmic principles of male and female. As they begin to interact in a more positive way, something new is created. Those who know the way to the future want that *something new* to occur now within humanity for humanity. This is the great mystery that is dawning at the edge of the enlightened human mind.

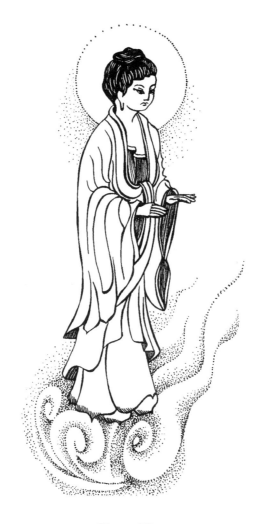

Kuan Yin
The Bodhisattva of Compassion

Chapter 3

The Ray Influence Hidden in the Rosary

Esotericism teaches that three great cosmic rays descend to humanity from the Trinity, the One expressing in three major forces and influencing all of life. We commonly think of these three forces as divine Will, divine Love and divine Intelligence. They are presented in many ways, the most familiar being the Trinity of the Father, the Son and the Holy Spirit. The esoteric tradition also uses the terms Will, Love-Wisdom and Active Intelligence for these three vital influences, or major rays of creation.

There is a stream of divine, life-giving energy that flows from the Creator to the creation.

Sometimes we call this great stream of life *grace;* often I call it the *light of the soul* or the *love of the soul.* To esotericists it is a spectrum of energies called the rays, analagous to rays of light or color. The wholeness is the complete spectrum of white light, like sunshine. If we separate this light into colors or purposes, we can describe and utilize the characteristics of the individual parts. Each segment of life has a point of identity on one ray. This is important to the structuring of each age, because each age brings a different blend of ray energies; thus the major influence of the age is determined. Slowly the ray influence remodels the life forms experiencing it.

The energy of the **first ray** is that of *Will,* empowering creation to a realization that a holy way exists: that Christ is, that the Hierarchy exists and that every human being contains a spark of God, charging life with ever-blooming, ever-unfolding reality. We will ourselves to work, to strive and to honor this great Life while doing our daily duty. At the same time, as we serve the highest Will we can perceive, we prepare ourselves for even greater work, greater will: "My will to Thy Will."

Love-Wisdom is the energy of the **second ray** and a necessity for walking the *Path of Initiation.* As devotion is lifted to aspiration, the emotional nature becomes a highly sensitive, beautiful vessel through which descending inspiration, spiritual truths, divine archetypes, blueprints and divine principles may find expression. The Path of Initiation unfolds within every son and daughter of God as they come to know their nature is love and their being is wise.

The **third ray** is often called *Active Intelligence,* or that which provides insights and experiences useful to the great life. The mental nature is extended to the higher, transcendental realities. Diversity of experience blends into the unique creation of those called *Masters* who, having mastered the physical, emotional and mental levels, identify with the spiritual and know that reality to be the true reality—all else is illusion. The third ray incorporates minor influences called the **fourth, fifth, sixth and seventh rays** which enrich Active Intelligence with omnipotence. Only the first three rays express at the highest level. These three energies begin the descent into matter and serve to guide the Soul back to the Source of Life through various initiations. Here the many facets synthesize into a great truth: "One Spirit, many gifts."

As we focus our attention on the mysteries of the rosary, we emphasize the Path of Initiation. This path of challenge and growth is really the coming to maturity within self that we might know the divine within. We acknowledge this as we speak of birthing the Christ-Within, or living in the Christ Presence. We come to know our spirituality—that the inner soul evolving into a high state of awareness is the purpose of enlight-

enment. The challenges one meets transform
the life and the response to it and ultimately
guide each aspirant to realizations of emerging
divinity hidden with form. The Path of Initiation is a centuries-old, symbolic name given to
the process of spiritual maturation we each seek
to master.

The rosary is especially beneficial for humanity
at this time of the Piscean-Aquarian Age change.
We have been building a vast ball of sixth ray devotional energy for more than 2,000 years. This
constitutes a great battery of devotion, or energy.
As we come under the influence of the Aquarian Age seventh ray, we can use this battery to
energize changes for the well-being of humanity.
The rosary is a seventh ray technique of mantras, prayers and invocations. Each time you say
the rosary, you utilize the energy of this ray to
advance the accumulation of devotional sixth
ray energy into new patterns of understanding.
For humanity this means transforming the old
in order to reveal the new. We are creating the
new mind, or New Jerusalem.

Chapter 4

The Rosary and Esoteric Christianity

As we approach the Aquarian Rosary, there are several important esoteric concepts that need fuller explanation and lead to a deeper understanding of the divine nature of humanity.

The ancient wisdom teaches that life is far greater than we have realized and that many teachers, saints and sages have evolved through the human path. In the beginning salutations of the rosary, we acknowledge all of these holy ones. In the esoteric Christian tradition these are usually referred to as the "Elder Brothers before the Throne." We are encouraged that others have traveled the quest and achieved; it is our goal to do likewise.

An *avatar* is a divine incarnation, an exalted being through whom the descending divinity may manifest on Earth to produce a desired effect upon humanity. An Eastern name for the returning avatar expected at this time is *Lord Maitreya*. The esoteric teaching says there is one avatar for each period, or epoch. We in the West call this expected one the *Christ*. Christ is a title, a principle and a great being.

The term *Father-Mother* is used throughout esoteric teachings as appropriate respect for both genders. The Creator, the One, spoke the Word and set into motion the lower world of duality, male and female. The statement or axiom "One becomes Three" refers to the One Creator flowing into the world of force and form. This idea is presented symbolically as the *Trinity*.

We may think of this as the Cosmic Oneness: "In the image of God he created him; male and female he created them."[1] One idea I like to use in understanding the Trinity is this: image first the Creator, second the creation and third the love that flows between them. This is expressed in Christianity as Father, Son and Holy Spirit.

The word *catholic* is Latin in origin and means universal. The planetary Christ came to declare a universal way. The early followers adopted the

---

1 Genesis 1:27, RSV

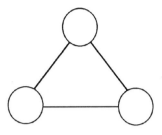

The Trinity

word to express their relationship with the universal teaching of Master Jesus, the Christ. When we say we believe in the holy catholic church, we acknowledge a universal approach. This does not pertain to the name of an institution but to the universality of the Christ's message and the body of believers that is ever expanding that message. We might remember, "In Christ there is neither male nor female; for you are all one in Christ Jesus."[1] This is truly catholic.

"Hail Mary, Mother of Earth" can be confusing unless we understand the Cosmic Feminine Principle that nourishes all of Life. The great feminine principle is always acknowledged in outstanding feminine lives to be held with respect and appreciation before humanity. Esoteric Christianity and the Mysteries of Isis taught respect and dignity for the female. In the East the feminine principle is represented by Kuan Yin.

---

1 Galatians 3:28, RSV

In his book *Bodhisattva of Compassion—The Mystical Tradition of Kuan Yin,*[1] John Blofeld writes:

> That Kuan Yin is actually seen with the eyes in one's head I doubt, but with the inner eye? Some who claim to have had this vision are people whose truthfulness is beyond question.

> Personally I think there was rather more to it than that, but there is a whole range of experience that would be difficult to classify as purely objective or subjective, so each of us has to interpret such phenomena in the way that seems best to him.... The key to the mystery was taught me by my teacher's teacher during a visit to Mongolia. There he came across images of Tara whom Mongols and Tibetans revere as a female emanation of Avalokita. Later on, my teacher, who loved to view collections of antique paintings, came upon several very old ones in which Kuan Yin was portrayed as being almost identical with Tara. In other words, for whatever reason, we Chinese decided to combine Avalokita and Tara into a sort of female Avalokita, whom we call Kuan Yin.

> Yogically she corresponds to an actual energy permanently latent in the mind; though it may be that the "forms" in which she is envisaged are deliberate human creations. Still, I think that the artists who

---

1 Boston: Shambhala, 1978

have best succeeded in capturing the magic
of those forms must have beheld them in
their meditations, for only in the stillness
of one-pointed contemplation is such perfection often revealed. Kuan Yin is unique
among the heavenly hierarchy in being ut-
terly free from pride or vengefulness and re-
luctant to punish even those to whom a
severe lesson would be salutary.

In the foreword of *Mother of the World*[1] we read:

> In the Hermetic Writings of old are found
> references to "the woman clothed with the
> Sun." Is this a symbol or a sublime Reality
> of the Higher World?

> Ancient religions, inspired by Messengers
> of the Planetary Hierarchy, accorded great
> reverence to the Feminine Principle in
> creation, the Mother aspect of Deity.

> The highest manifestation of this Femi-
> nine Principle has been called by many
> names, among them, Mother of the Uni-
> verse, World Mother, Isis, Istar and Sophia.
> To the Gnostic Christians she was known
> as the Holy Spirit, one of the Divine Triad;
> but ecclesiastical Christianity has regarded
> the Holy Trinity as entirely masculine,
> thus depriving its adherents of a sublime
> and ennobling concept.

To say "Holy Mary, Mother of Gods" can be really hard when we are also saying we believe

1 Agni Yoga Society, 319 W. 107th St., New York, NY,
  1956

there is one God, Creator of all life. The Old
Testament states, "I say, You are Gods, and all
of you are children of the Most High."[1] And
again in the New Testament Jesus said, "Is it not
written in your law, I said, You are gods?"[2] The
Mother, the feminine principle of life, would
raise us into the human Gods we truly are. We
are reminded that we too are Gods-in-the-
process-of-becoming, even as Master Jesus became the Christ.

We call upon the Lord Jesus to help us. We acknowledge Him as the guru or master of the
Christian way and remember His promise that
He is always available to us as we follow His
path of ascent. The disciple knows that when he
invokes help in the holy name of the Wayshower, it will come. "Ask and ye shall receive."
In these words we are asking.

The Structure of the Aquarian Rosary

To say the rosary, a few short prayers are offered
as an introduction. Then a pattern of ten repetitive prayers called a *decade* (pronounced dek'ud)
is established as the mysteries are contemplated.

Mysteries and secrets are not synonymous. A
secret is something that one person knows and,
when shared, another knows as well. A *mystery*
is a realization that slowly dawns upon one as

---

1 Psalm 82:6, RSV
2 John 10:34, AV

s/he contemplates. As one comes time and again to the spiritual mysteries, the inner meaning becomes known to the meditator.

In each set of mysteries we see the areas of human life to be transformed as the mystical Christ-Within stands revealed. The mysteries acknowledge the hidden, little-understood energies that direct the inner life. The chalice, alive with fire, purifies all that enters the Light. The term *chalice* is used for the open high consciousness that can receive inspiration, vision and straight knowledge from the Christ, the Godhead or the Dharma Light. The divine expression may be called by many names, but all traditions are trying to acknowledge *the holy contact*. The higher planes are the home of the Soul—here all is unveiled.

The one-of-a-kind prayers represent the uniqueness of the individual as well as the oneness of God when all is realized. Just as the one is significant, the other numbers reveal their hidden influences as we study. The power of ten is that of masculine and feminine energies learning to work in perfect harmony with properly balanced energy. We begin as individuals having much to learn; we become balanced co-workers with God in whom "all things are possible."

The number five is important in light of the five decades of beads that are used in each set of mysteries of the rosary. Five is seen as the number of humanity, as the union of two (feminine) and three (masculine). The number does not imply harmony but, as a number of life, it is ever seeking that which is higher than it knows.

The five decades of each set represent the preparation of the physical, emotional, mental, spiritual and social levels of our lives to receive the inspiration, higher laws and, later, the commands. The five groupings of ten beads draw our attention to our own transformation from lesser will, the one (independent and alone) to the tenth (balanced within self and transformed) ready now to co-work with higher will and higher worlds. Each series of five decades also represents areas of concentration for one's inner development. These areas are the initiations taken in the human path of experience.

The first five decades of the rosary are known as *The Joyful Mysteries*. Here we acknowledge and invoke the ray one aspect of Will. We are reminded of the will we need to make progress. As we begin the spiritual journey, we become candidates for the Path, laying a foundation of alignment with the Will of the Creator in the shaping of the physical life.

The second five decades, *The Sorrowful Mysteries*, invoke the ray two aspect of Love-Wisdom as we seek to understand the Path of Initiation. Our attention is called to the task the aspirant has if s/he would understand life in the physical, material world. Acknowledging sorrow and coming to understand its limiting nature, one sets one's sights on freedom.

The third five decades are *The Glorious Mysteries*, which present the concepts of third ray energy, or Active Intelligence. The Glorious Mysteries often seem misnamed and beyond our comprehension. Here our contemplative work is directed to the hard-to-understand other-world interactions after the death of Master Jesus. We are challenged to believe that the higher worlds can open and phenomena not common to physical life can occur. Our ability to penetrate into the *Cloud of Knowable Things* must develop for us to go beyond faith and *know*. We want to experience the divine realizations. We would know the Truth and be set free of our own disbelief. The challenge of the infinite presents itself to the finite, and we struggle to expand to the edge of mind.

A complete rosary is rarely said. To do so, one would circle the common rosary three times and include the Joyful, Sorrowful and Glorious Mysteries all. Usually only one of the three sets of prayers is offered at a time.

Ideals contemplated in the mysteries guide us to the proper use of Will, the awareness of Love-Wisdom and ultimately into right-relationship to Higher Intelligence. Situations used in the rosary for contemplation are stories dear to the Christian tradition. These preserve the parables, the life of Master Jesus and the little understood mystical happenings of the Christ. Ideas to be contemplated also call to our attention the qualities of the higher nature we must develop as we travel the Path of Initiation called the Christian Way.

With the dawning of the Aquarian Age, we will find a new appreciation of the mystery tradition. We will see the lonely and often reclusive aspirant of the past become the world server of today. This one-made-ready is anxious to be deeply involved in co-working, brotherhood-sisterhood, acknowledgement of a universal God and respect for each path. We are reminded of the old comment, "The Masters dwell in peace as the disciples quarrel." As we gain an understanding of the mystic way in the Aquarian Age, we will find the All-Pervading Presence uniting the family of humanity.

Traditionally, prayer beads have been used to help one contemplate sacred thoughts—to keep one tracking, almost without thought. The prayers of the intellectual mind rapidly become the mantras of inner contemplation as the fingers slide over the beads. Physical words are spoken as the mind explores the inner realities of spiritual life. The heart filled with devotion energizes the outer life with deep caring. Chanting, movement and contemplation are linked together in the great mystery technique of mantra meditation. The total brain utilization energizes the transformational process that the fervent heart seeks.

Let us now experience the Aquarian Rosary together.

Part II

THE TECHNIQUE

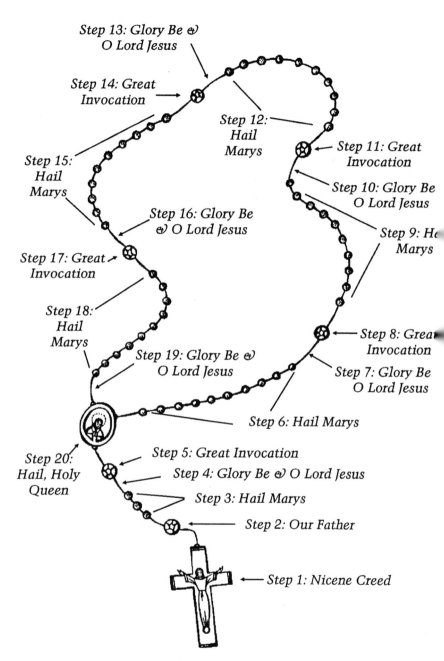

The Aquarian Rosary

Introduction to Part II

The three rosaries presented in this section are designed to be used in actual ritualistic practice by the reader. I encourage you to participate in group use of the rosaries; however, it is perfectly appropriate for you to say the rosaries alone if you wish.

For persons wanting a daily practice, Monday and Thursday are historically the days on which the Joyful is said. The Sorrowful is offered on Tuesdays and Fridays, and the Glorious Mysteries are prayed on Wednesday and Saturday.

Saturday is the day that in recent apparitions (Fatima, for example) Mother Mary has asked that the rosary be said. Therefore, the most common way of offering the rosary is to say one set of prayers as a regular practice on Saturdays. Persons usually alternate between the Joyful, the Sorrowful and the Glorious from week to week. It is customary in the Catholic tradition for rosaries to be said for special intentions and for individuals in need. A regular practice is to say the rosary for individuals who have made their transition, as an invocation of grace on behalf of the deceased.

Nearly all prayer work is preceded by a sign or movement signifying the nature of the work to the subconscious, or basic self. Some persons kneel to pray and bow their heads or fold their hands in prayer position. Any of these practices becomes a signal to the inner nature that one is shifting consciousness and turning the attention away from things of the outer to do inner work.

To begin, then, decide what your own signal is to be. I happen to like making the sign of the cross on myself with the rosary. The sign of the cross is an old mystical sign of the opening of the chakra centers for the inflow of grace. Many persons are more comfortable folding their palms together and bowing their head in a sign of greeting to God. Whatever you choose, it signals your lower nature to settle down and prepare for spiritual work.

I have listed this preparatory practice in the technique with a reference to the cross of the Risen Christ. The Risen Christ will become the Christ most used on the cross during the Aquarian Age as we move away from the crucifix, the symbol of Christ which served us in the Piscean Age. The crucifix symbolized the suffering and sacrificial service offered by Master Jesus. We will now begin to move from the sorrowful symbolism of Good Friday to the joy-filled symbolism of Easter morn. Humanity will leave behind its preoccupation with suffering; instead, it will desire to rise higher into the awareness of the message delivered by Master Jesus, the Christ.

In the new rosary technique, we begin to get acquainted with the mysteries of the Christ, offered to a humanity who would "do the work." If you have a favorite rosary that bears the crucified Christ and you wish to continue using it, feel free to do so. However, you may choose to obtain a Risen Christ cross and put it on your rosary in place of the crucifix. Such crosses are available in any number of places, including the Sparrow Hawk Village Gift Shop (P.O. Box 1274, Tahlequah, Oklahoma 74465).

The technique is set up with a leader offering the salutations and the audience/congregation/group doing the response. If you are doing the rosary alone, simply ignore the textual distinction between leader and response and say both parts yourself. The rosary is a chant as well as a prayer, so it lends itself to the leader-response style. Down through the ages, however, it has also been a very important silent chant/meditation/prayer technique for the individual; and it will continue to contribute to our lives in this way.

Directions are given for the steps as one moves through them. The illustration of the rosary above allows one to become acquainted with the beads and placement of fingers used for the procedure.

Think of the technique of the rosary as a shift from outer awareness and study to inner awareness, prayer, seed thought meditation and movement of fingers on the beads. This is the intense focusing that is needed for reprogramming of self that is the work of Mantra Yoga. We are using the prayers as mantras to help us know our identity with the divine feminine of our desire.

A complete rosary comprises three trips around the full circle of beads. When the particular set of mysteries you choose for a single session is completed, you will have circled the beads one time (one-third of a complete rosary). This is called *one circlet*. One circlet is commonly called a rosary, but you now know that in fact three sets make up the whole. On occasion you will see a particularly long set of beads that reaches to near the knee, usually worn by a brother, priest or nun. This is a set that has three of the regular size strands of beads together: a complete rosary.

As you say the rosary, do not attempt to make each word clear and distinct. The words will begin to take on a cadence, and this will allow the chanting effect to emerge. Relax into the cadence. As you do this, you will begin to experience the powerful effect of energy work; and the deeper meaning of the ritual of the rosary will become apparent.

You are now ready to proceed.

Chapter 5

The Joyful Mysteries

This rosary has been prayerfully inspired by love of Our Lady and an understanding of the Power of the Spoken Holy Word in awakening human minds to the Light, Love and Spiritual Power available to humanity. May the speaking of these Holy Mantras invoke the power of Good into each life, uplift and stimulate open minds and build a heart center that can utilize the Lots of Vital Energies of the unfolding human soul.

Let us begin:[1] *(Looking at the cross of the Risen Christ on the pendulum of the rosary, some may wish to kiss the cross or cross themselves)*

1st STEP:

Salutations to The Masters of Wisdom, the Elder Brothers of Humanity.

Response: OM

Salutations to The Lord Maitreya, The Christ, the Head of Hierarchy, Teacher of Angels and of Humanity.

Response: OM

Salutations to The Christ, the path between Humanity, Hierarchy and the Fiery Mind of God.

Response: OM

The Nicene Creed *(said on the Cross of the Risen Christ)*

We believe in one God, the Father-Mother Almighty, maker of heaven and earth, of all that is, seen and unseen; We believe in our Lord, Jesus Christ, the Holy Son of God, eternally begotten of the Father-Mother, God from God, Light from Light, true God from true God, begotten, not made, of one Being with the Father-Mother Almighty through

---

1 The rosaries are performed in a leader–response style. Within each Step, boldface text indicates phrases spoken by the leader, and normal text designates the group response.

whom all things were made. For us and for
our salvation Christ came down from
heaven, by the power of the Holy Spirit became incarnate through the Virgin Mary, and
was made man, was crucified under Pontius
Pilate, suffered death and was buried. On the
third day he arose in accordance with the
Scriptures; he ascended into heaven and assumed his rightful place of service. He will
come again in glory to judge the living and
the dead, and his kingdom will have no end.

We believe in the Holy Spirit, the giver of life,
who proceeds from the Father-Mother and
the Son. S/He is worshiped and glorified.[1] S/He has spoken through the Prophets.
We believe in one holy catholic and apostolic
church. We acknowledge one baptism for the
forgiveness of sins, the resurrection of the
dead and the life of the world to come. Amen.

2nd STEP:

We join together in saying the Our Father
(said on the first bead)

Our Father, Who is throughout the Universe,
Let Your Name be set apart
Come Your Kingdom
Let Your delight be in earth
As it is throughout the Universe.

---

1 The early church used "He" in the Nicene Creed, but
often spoke of the Holy Spirit as "She." We have chosen
to respect both.

Give us bread for our necessities today
And forgive us our offenses as we have for-
    given our offenders.
And do not let us enter into materialism
But set us free from error.
Because yours is the Kingdom and the Power
    and the Song from age to age sealed in faith-
    fulness and truth. Amen.
    *(Aramaic Translation of the model prayer
    better known as the "Lord's Prayer")*

3rd STEP:

Three Hail Marys *(said on the set of 3 beads
as we invoke the Light, Love and Spiritual
Power of our unfolding soul)*

**Hail Mary, Mother of Earth, the Lords love
Thee. Blessed are You throughout the Universe and blessed are the Children of Humanity.**
Holy Mary, Mother of Gods, nourish us with
wisdom and inspire us through the experience of life and death. Amen.

4th STEP:

One Glory Be *(said on wire before large
single bead)*

**Glory be to the Father-Mother and to the Son
and to the Holy Spirit.**
As it was in the beginning, is now and ever
shall be, world without end. Amen.

O, Lord Jesus, forgive us our errors and aid us in our quest.
Lead all souls to Light and Love, especially those most in need of your mercy. Amen.

5th STEP: *(said on large single bead)*

We focus on the power of the first ray, Will.
It is the will of the Creator that all life know the joy of Oneness. The First Joyful Mystery is the Annunciation. The angel comes to Mary. He greets her, "Hail, full of grace, the Lord is with thee. Blessed art thou among women." The esoteric understanding requires that we build humility within our nature as we are accepted into the company of the spiritually dedicated.

We join together in the saying of the Great Invocation.

From the point of Light within the mind
    of God
Let Light stream forth into the minds of men.
Let Light descend on Earth.

From the point of Love within the Heart
    of God
Let Love stream forth into the hearts of men.
May Christ return to Earth.

From the centre where the Will of God
    is known
Let purpose guide the little wills of men—
The purpose which the Masters know
    and serve.

From the centre which we call the race
of men
Let the plan of Love and Light work out.
And may it seal the door where evil dwells.

Let Light and Love and Power restore the
Plan on Earth.

6th STEP:

Ten Hail Marys as we contemplate the importance of humility. "Be it done unto me according to Thy Will"; humility accepts the divine pattern.

Hail Mary, Mother of Earth, the Lords love Thee. Blessed are You throughout the Universe and blessed are the Children of Humanity.

Holy Mary, Mother of Gods, nourish us with wisdom and inspire us through the experience of life and death. Amen.

7th STEP: *(said on wire before large single bead)*

Glory be to the Father-Mother and to the Son and to the Holy Spirit.

As it was in the beginning, is now and ever shall be, world without end. Amen.

O, Lord Jesus, forgive us our errors and aid us in our quest.

Lead all souls to Light and Love, especially those most in need of your mercy. Amen.

8th STEP: *(said on large single bead)*

The Second Joyful Mystery is the Visitation.
Mary goes to visit Elizabeth and assists her before the births of the holy children. We contemplate the esoteric teaching of service to the world. We bring our will to serve. As we realize our interlocking bonds, service becomes our reason for being.

We join together in the saying of the Great Invocation.

From the point of Light within the mind
    of God
Let Light stream forth into the minds of men.
Let Light descend on Earth.

From the point of Love within the Heart
    of God
Let Love stream forth into the hearts of men.
May Christ return to Earth.

From the centre where the Will of God
    is known
Let purpose guide the little wills of men—
The purpose which the Masters know
    and serve.

From the centre which we call the race
    of men
Let the plan of Love and Light work out.
And may it seal the door where evil dwells.

Let Light and Love and Power restore the
    Plan on Earth.

9th STEP:

> Ten Hail Marys as we contemplate Service to the world. We grow in understanding of the Master's commandments: "Love one another, serve one another."
>
> **Hail Mary, Mother of Earth, the Lords love Thee. Blessed are You throughout the Universe and blessed are the Children of Humanity.**
>
> Holy Mary, Mother of Gods, nourish us with wisdom and inspire us through the experience of life and death. Amen.

10th STEP: *(said on wire before large single bead)*

> **Glory be to the Father-Mother and to the Son and to the Holy Spirit.**
>
> As it was in the beginning, is now and ever shall be, world without end. Amen.
>
> **O, Lord Jesus, forgive us our errors and aid us in our quest.**
>
> Lead all souls to Light and Love, especially those most in need of your mercy. Amen.

11th STEP: *(said on large single bead)*

> **The Third Joyful Mystery is the Nativity.**
>
> Sometimes called privacy, sometimes called poverty, we come to know in the privacy of our secret ponderings of life that no material riches can bring enlightenment. We are alone

with our real worth. We are destined to grow
and overcome every obstacle as we become
children of Light.

**We join together in the saying of the Great
Invocation.**

From the point of Light within the mind
   of God
Let Light stream forth into the minds of men.
Let Light descend on Earth.

From the point of Love within the Heart
   of God
Let Love stream forth into the hearts of men.
May Christ return to Earth.

From the centre where the Will of God
   is known
Let purpose guide the little wills of men—
The purpose which the Masters know
   and serve.

From the centre which we call the race
   of men
Let the plan of Love and Light work out.
And may it seal the door where evil dwells.

Let Light and Love and Power restore the
   Plan on Earth.

12th STEP:

**Ten Hail Marys as we contemplate privacy of
inner thoughts. This is especially important
as we realize "thoughts are things." We will
ourselves to support the positive and to be a
blessing to the environment.**

Hail Mary, Mother of Earth, the Lords love Thee. Blessed are You throughout the Universe and blessed are the Children of Humanity.

Holy Mary, Mother of Gods, nourish us with wisdom and inspire us through the experience of life and death. Amen.

13th STEP: *(said on wire before large single bead)*

Glory be to the Father-Mother and to the Son and to the Holy Spirit.

As it was in the beginning, is now and ever shall be, world without end. Amen.

O, Lord Jesus, forgive us our errors and aid us in our quest.

Lead all souls to Light and Love, especially those most in need of your mercy. Amen.

14th STEP: *(said on large single bead)*

The Fourth Joyful Mystery is the Presentation in the Temple.

Here Jesus demonstrates his understanding of Spiritual Law. Each of us is challenged in life to demonstrate our understanding and obedience to spiritual law. We realize we belong not to the personality but to the world of souls.

We join together in saying the Great Invocation.

From the point of Light within the mind
     of God
Let Light stream forth into the minds of men.
Let Light descend on Earth.

From the point of Love within the Heart
     of God
Let Love stream forth into the hearts of men.
May Christ return to Earth.

From the centre where the Will of God
     is known
Let purpose guide the little wills of men—
The purpose which the Masters know
     and serve.

From the centre which we call the race
     of men
Let the plan of Love and Light work out.
And may it seal the door where evil dwells.

Let Light and Love and Power restore the
     Plan on Earth.

15th STEP:

Ten Hail Marys as we contemplate the importance of spiritual laws and the importance of will if we would be obedient to the Laws of the Universe.

Hail Mary, Mother of Earth, the Lords love Thee. Blessed are You throughout the Universe and blessed are the Children of Humanity.

Holy Mary, Mother of Gods, nourish us with wisdom and inspire us through the experience of life and death. Amen.

16th STEP: *(said on wire before large single bead)*

Glory be to the Father-Mother and to the Son and to the Holy Spirit.

As it was in the beginning, is now and ever shall be, world without end. Amen.

O, Lord Jesus, forgive us our errors and aid us in our quest.

Lead all souls to Light and Love, especially those most in need of your mercy. Amen

17th STEP: *(said on large single bead)*

The Fifth Joyful Mystery is the Finding of Jesus in the Temple.

The esoteric teaching reminds us, "We must be about our Father's business", or our soul purpose. As we come to know, we are held accountable for our choices. Personality becomes the chalice for the Soul.

We join together in saying The Great Invocation.

From the point of Light within the mind
    of God
Let Light stream forth into the minds of men.
Let Light descend on Earth.

From the point of Love within the Heart
of God
Let Love stream forth into the hearts of men.
May Christ return to Earth.

From the centre where the Will of God
is known
Let purpose guide the little wills of men—
The purpose which the Masters know
and serve.

From the centre which we call the race
of men
Let the plan of Love and Light work out.
And may it seal the door where evil dwells.

Let Light and Love and Power restore the
Plan on Earth.

18th STEP:

Ten Hail Marys as we contemplate what we detect as our purpose in life—why we have entered into the world of form. We seek to draw more soul awareness into the physical world of matter. We contemplate listening inwardly to realize our reason for being. We will the Holy Will in our lives.

Hail Mary, Mother of Earth, the Lords love Thee. Blessed are You throughout the Universe and blessed are the Children of Humanity.

Holy Mary, Mother of Gods, nourish us with wisdom and inspire us through the experience of life and death. Amen

19th STEP: *(said on wire before holy medal)*

Glory be to the Father-Mother and to the Son and to the Holy Spirit.

As it was in the beginning, is now and ever shall be, world without end. Amen.

O, Lord Jesus, forgive us our errors and aid us in our quest.

Lead all souls to Light and Love, especially those most in need of your mercy. Amen.

20th STEP: *(said on the holy medal)*

Hail, Holy Queen, Mother of Mercy, our Life, our Sweetness and our Hope, to You do we turn our hearts as the awakening Children of Eve; to You do we send up our prayers, invoking Your Love.

Turn, then, most gracious Advocate, your eyes of mercy toward us, and after this, our period of growth, open to us the kingdom of souls. O clement, O loving, O sweet Mother Mary!

Pray for us, O Holy Mother of Gods, that we may experience the promises of Christ as was willed for us from the beginning. Amen.

This concludes the Joyful Mysteries and the first rosary.

Chapter 6

The Sorrowful Mysteries

The Sorrowful Mysteries are to aid us in understanding the "cause of sorrow." Buddha gave us the Noble Truths and the Eight-Fold Path to help us understand the nature of sorrow and how to develop the wisdom needed to free ourselves. The Christ embodied the Love principle that we might care for others unconditionally. The second set of mysteries of the rosary is called The Sorrowful Mysteries and works with the ray two energy of Love-Wisdom. As we contemplate these parables, we realize the development of the Christ-Within. Love-Wisdom is necessary to walk the Path of Initiation.

Let us begin[1] *(Looking at cross of the Risen Christ on the pendulum of the rosary, some may wish to kiss the cross or cross themselves)*

1st STEP:

> **Salutations to The Masters of Wisdom, the Elder Brothers of Humanity.**
>
> Response: OM
>
> **Salutations to The Lord Maitreya, The Christ, the Head of Hierarchy, Teacher of Angels and of Humanity.**
>
> Response: OM
>
> **Salutations to The Christ, the path between Humanity, Hierarchy and the Fiery Mind of God.**
>
> Response: OM
>
> **The Nicene Creed** *(said on the Cross of the Risen Christ)*
>
> **We believe in one God, the Father-Mother Almighty, maker of heaven and earth, of all that is, seen and unseen; We believe in our Lord, Jesus Christ, the Holy Son of God, eternally begotten of the Father-Mother, God from God, Light from Light, true God from true God, begotten, not made, of one Being with the Father-Mother Almighty through**

---

1 The rosaries are performed in a leader–response style. Within each Step, boldface text indicates phrases spoken by the leader, and normal text designates the group response.

whom all things were made. For us and for our salvation Christ came down from heaven, by the power of the Holy Spirit became incarnate through the Virgin Mary, and was made man, was crucified under Pontius Pilate, suffered death and was buried. On the third day he arose in accordance with the Scriptures; he ascended into heaven and assumed his rightful place of service. He will come again in glory to judge the living and the dead, and his kingdom will have no end.

We believe in the Holy Spirit, the giver of life, who proceeds from the Father-Mother and the Son. S/He is worshiped and glorified.[1] S/He has spoken through the Prophets. We believe in one holy catholic and apostolic church. We acknowledge one baptism for the forgiveness of sins, the resurrection of the dead and the life of the world to come. Amen.

2nd STEP:

We join together in saying the Our Father *(said on the first bead)*

Our Father, Who is throughout the Universe,

Let Your Name be set apart
Come Your Kingdom
Let Your delight be in earth
As it is throughout the Universe.

---

1 The early church used "He" in the Nicene Creed, but often spoke of the Holy Spirit as "She." We have chosen to respect both.

Give us bread for our necessities today
And forgive us our offenses as we have for-
   given our offenders.
And do not let us enter into materialism
But set us free from error.
Because yours is the Kingdom and the Power
   and the Song from age to age sealed in faith-
   fulness and truth. Amen.
*(Aramaic Translation of the model prayer
   better known as the "Lord's Prayer")*

3rd STEP:

Three Hail Marys *(said on the set of 3 beads
as we invoke the Light, Love and Spiritual
Power of our unfolding soul)*

**Hail Mary, Mother of Earth, the Lords love
Thee. Blessed are You throughout the Universe and blessed are the Children of Humanity.**

Holy Mary, Mother of Gods, nourish us with
wisdom and inspire us through the experience of life and death. Amen.

4th STEP:

One Glory Be *(said on wire before large
single bead)*

**Glory be to the Father-Mother and to the Son
and to the Holy Spirit.**

As it was in the beginning, is now and ever
shall be, world without end. Amen.

O, Lord Jesus, forgive us our errors and aid us in our quest.
Lead all souls to Light and Love, especially those most in need of your mercy. Amen.

5th STEP: *(said on large single bead)*

The First Sorrowful Mystery is the Agony in the Garden.
While it acknowledges Thy Will/not mine, there is also the underlying realization that the Higher has a reason for all actions. Nothing happens without a cause. There are no accidents, only ways and means of calling us to a higher awareness. The Love-Wisdom of God has a purpose in our lives and we can trust that Love and that Wisdom to bring forth from within us more than we can see.

We join together in the saying of the Great Invocation.
From the point of Light within the mind
    of God
Let Light stream forth into the minds of men.
Let Light descend on Earth.

From the point of Love within the Heart
    of God
Let Love stream forth into the hearts of men.
May Christ return to Earth.

From the centre where the Will of God
    is known
Let purpose guide the little wills of men—

The purpose which the Masters know
and serve.

From the centre which we call the race
of men
Let the plan of Love and Light work out.
And may it seal the door where evil dwells.

Let Light and Love and Power restore the
Plan on Earth.

6th STEP:

**Ten Hail Marys as we contemplate the Love
that sustains us, the Lots Of Vital Energy of
the Soul, as we become wise enough to see a
Higher Plan.**

**Hail Mary, Mother of Earth, the Lords love
Thee. Blessed are You throughout the Universe and blessed are the Children of Humanity.**

Holy Mary, Mother of Gods, nourish us with
wisdom and inspire us through the experience of life and death. Amen

7th STEP: *(said on wire before large single bead)*

**Glory be to the Father-Mother and to the Son
and to the Holy Spirit.**

As it was in the beginning, is now and ever
shall be, world without end. Amen.

**O, Lord Jesus, forgive us our errors and aid us
in our quest.**

Lead all souls to Light and Love, especially those most in need of your mercy. Amen.

8th STEP: *(said on large single bead)*

The Second Sorrowful Mystery is Master Jesus Scourged in the Temple.

This painful scene reminds us of the pain and suffering of the human condition—how cruel we are to one another, forgetting that each is a child of God. The path to the Light within is difficult, and as we become sensitive, we begin to release our identity with the physical nature and build our identity with the spiritual. Even the seed suffers as it breaks through to let the sprout within come to life. The nature of the physical is to bounce between ecstasy and pain. Embrace wisdom to be free.

We join together in the saying of the Great Invocation.

From the point of Light within the mind
     of God
Let Light stream forth into the minds of men.
Let Light descend on Earth.

From the point of Love within the Heart
     of God
Let Love stream forth into the hearts of men.
May Christ return to Earth.

From the centre where the Will of God
     is known
Let purpose guide the little wills of men—

The purpose which the Masters know
and serve.

From the centre which we call the race
of men
Let the plan of Love and Light work out.
And may it seal the door where evil dwells.

Let Light and Love and Power restore the
Plan on Earth.

9th STEP:

Ten Hail Marys as we contemplate the Wisdom needed to see the outcome of physical suffering about us. We release our attachments and addictions and through detachment, dispassion and disidentification find our way to a higher perspective.

Hail Mary, Mother of Earth, the Lords love Thee. Blessed are You throughout the Universe and blessed are the Children of Humanity.

Holy Mary, Mother of Gods, nourish us with wisdom and inspire us through the experience of life and death. Amen.

10th STEP: *(said on wire before large single bead)*

Glory be to the Father-Mother and to the Son and to the Holy Spirit.

As it was in the beginning, is now and ever shall be, world without end. Amen.

O, Lord Jesus, forgive us our errors and aid us in our quest.

Lead all souls to Light and Love, especially those most in need of your mercy. Amen.

11th STEP: *(said on large single bead)*

The Third Sorrowful Mystery is Master Jesus Crowned with Thorns.

Each initiate will pierce through to the mental world and in so doing will be challenged. Thus the crown is won. Courage is a must for the spiritual aspirant. Courage builds the Heart Center which can anchor the positive energies of the soul in the face of the just or the unjust.

We join together in the saying of the Great Invocation.

From the point of Light within the mind
    of God
Let Light stream forth into the minds of men.
Let Light descend on Earth.

From the point of Love within the Heart
    of God
Let Love stream forth into the hearts of men.
May Christ return to Earth.

From the centre where the Will of God
    is known
Let purpose guide the little wills of men—
The purpose which the Masters know
    and serve.

From the centre which we call the race
 of men
Let the plan of Love and Light work out.
And may it seal the door where evil dwells.
Let Light and Love and Power restore the
 Plan on Earth.

12th STEP:

**Ten Hail Marys as we contemplate the pain
of seeing a way others do not see. We realize
we are to lift ourselves out of the emotional
pain and suffering and become wise that we
may assist with the transformation of the
pain-filled world into a renewed Garden of
Eden. We seek the love and wisdom needed
to be the wise stewards using well the oppor-
tunity of physical life.**

**Hail Mary, Mother of Earth, the Lords love
Thee. Blessed are You throughout the Universe and blessed are the Children of Humanity.**

Holy Mary, Mother of Gods, nourish us with
wisdom and inspire us through the experience of life and death. Amen.

13th STEP: *(said on wire before large single
bead)*

**Glory be to the Father-Mother and to the Son
and to the Holy Spirit.**

As it was in the beginning, is now and ever
shall be, world without end. Amen.

O, Lord Jesus, forgive us our errors and aid us in our quest.

Lead all souls to Light and Love, especially those most in need of your mercy. Amen.

14th STEP: *(said on large single bead)*

The The Fourth Sorrowful Mystery is Master Jesus Carrying the Cross.

This scene has encouraged the mystics for centuries as each also carries the cross of life. We are challenged by the strengths and weaknesses of our own nature as we would bring to balance the forces of spirit and matter, of heart and mind. The cross is overcome and we are freed through the transformational power of the Heart Center. We are challenged to build patience and endurance as we go about our lives, doing the disciplines of our spiritual practice.

We join together in the saying of the Great Invocation.

From the point of Light within the mind
    of God
Let Light stream forth into the minds of men.
Let Light descend on Earth.

From the point of Love within the Heart
    of God
Let Love stream forth into the hearts of men.
May Christ return to Earth.

From the centre where the Will of God
    is known

Let purpose guide the little wills of men—
The purpose which the Masters know
   and serve.
From the centre which we call the race
   of men
Let the plan of Love and Light work out.
And may it seal the door where evil dwells.
Let Light and Love and Power restore the
   Plan on Earth.

15th STEP:

Ten Hail Marys as we contemplate the patience and endurance needed on the Path of Initiation. We continue with dedication the Path we walk. Patience is realized and endurance comes. The awakening one goes about the world, doing well the work at hand that greater service may come.

Hail Mary, Mother of Earth, the Lords love Thee. Blessed are You throughout the Universe and blessed are the Children of Humanity.

Holy Mary, Mother of Gods, nourish us with wisdom and inspire us through the experience of life and death. Amen.

16th STEP: *(said on wire before large single bead)*

Glory be to the Father-Mother and to the Son and to the Holy Spirit.

As it was in the beginning, is now and ever shall be, world without end. Amen.

O, Lord Jesus, forgive us our errors and aid us in our quest.

Lead all souls to Light and Love, especially those most in need of your mercy. Amen

17th STEP: *(said on large single bead)*

The Fifth Sorrowful Mystery is Master Jesus Dying on the Cross.

The victory over the world of duality is won. Holy Ones, to complete their work in the world of the lesser, must give their life for something worthwhile. We remember Master Jesus as the Wayshower who demonstrates for the Christian way that the gaining of the spiritual life is worth giving all. The Crucifixion stands before each of us, that we may stand as an adept, strong in our own right. We die to the lesser to become the greater.

We join together in the saying of the Great Invocation.

From the point of Light within the mind
    of God
Let Light stream forth into the minds of men.
Let Light descend on Earth.

From the point of Love within the Heart
    of God
Let Love stream forth into the hearts of men.
May Christ return to Earth.

From the centre where the Will of God
   is known
Let purpose guide the little wills of men—
The purpose which the Masters know
   and serve.

From the centre which we call the race
   of men
Let the plan of Love and Light work out.
And may it seal the door where evil dwells.

Let Light and Love and Power restore the
   Plan on Earth.

18th STEP:

Ten Hail Marys as we contemplate the challenges that seek to slow us on the Path of Initiation. We realize that hard steps lead to a Great Goal. We rededicate ourselves to meeting our challenges well, taking the tests and loving the Holy Ones who have gone before us to show us the way.

Hail Mary, Mother of Earth, the Lords love Thee. Blessed are You throughout the Universe and blessed are the Children of Humanity.

Holy Mary, Mother of Gods, nourish us with wisdom and inspire us through the experience of life and death. Amen

19th STEP: *(said on wire before holy medal)*

Glory be to the Father-Mother and to the Son and to the Holy Spirit.

As it was in the beginning, is now and ever shall be, world without end. Amen.

O, Lord Jesus, forgive our errors and aid us in our quest.

Lead all souls to Light and Love, especially those most in need of your mercy. Amen.

20th STEP: *(said on the holy medal)*

Hail, Holy Queen, Mother of Mercy, our Life, our Sweetness and our Hope, to You do we turn our hearts as the awakening Children of Eve; to You do we send up our prayers, invoking Your love.

Turn, then, most gracious Advocate, your eyes of mercy toward us, and after this, our period of growth, open to us the kingdom of souls. O clement, O loving, O sweet Mother Mary!

Pray for us, O Holy Mother of Gods, that we may experience the promises of Christ as was willed for us from the beginning. Amen.

This concludes the sorrowful Mysteries and ends the second rosary.

Chapter 7

The Glorious Mysteries

The Glorious Mysteries share with us the impact of ray three, Active Intelligence, for the initiate enters into ideas and teachings that far surpass our everyday understanding. Here we are challenged to grow into a mystical attunement to higher realities. Our limited mind must release its hold to experience Divine Mind. We move from limitation to fullness within the Light of Christ.

Let us begin:[1] *(Looking at the cross of the Risen Christ on the pendulum of the rosary some may wish to kiss the cross or cross themselves)*

1st STEP:

> **Salutations to The Masters of Wisdom, the Elder Brothers of Humanity.**
>
> Response: OM
>
> **Salutations to The Lord Maitreya, The Christ, the Head of Hierarchy, Teacher of Angels and of Humanity.**
>
> Response: OM
>
> **Salutations to The Christ, the path between Humanity, Hierarchy and the Fiery Mind of God.**
>
> Response: OM
>
> **The Nicene Creed** *(said on the Cross of the Risen Christ)*
>
> **We believe in one God, the Father-Mother Almighty, maker of heaven and earth, of all that is, seen and unseen; We believe in our Lord, Jesus Christ, the Holy Son of God, eternally begotten of the Father-Mother, God from God, Light from Light, true God from true God, begotten, not made, of one Being with the Father-Mother Almighty through**

---

1 The rosaries are performed in a leader–response style. Within each Step, boldface text indicates phrases spoken by the leader, and normal text designates the group response.

whom all things were made. For us and for our salvation Christ came down from heaven, by the power of the Holy Spirit became incarnate through the Virgin Mary, and was made man, was crucified under Pontius Pilate, suffered death and was buried. On the third day he arose in accordance with the Scriptures; he ascended into heaven and assumed his rightful place of service. He will come again in glory to judge the living and the dead, and his kingdom will have no end.

We believe in the Holy Spirit, the giver of life, who proceeds from the Father-Mother and the Son. S/He is worshiped and glorified.[1] S/He has spoken through the Prophets. We believe in one holy catholic and apostolic church. We acknowledge one baptism for the forgiveness of sins, the resurrection of the dead and the life of the world to come. Amen.

2nd STEP:

We join together in saying the Our Father *(said on the first bead)*

Our Father, Who is throughout the Universe,
Let Your Name be set apart
Come Your Kingdom
Let Your delight be in earth
As it is throughout the Universe.

---

1 The early church used "He" in the Nicene Creed, but often spoke of the Holy Spirit as "She." We have chosen to respect both.

Give us bread for our necessities today
And forgive us our offenses as we have for-
  given our offenders.
And do not let us enter into materialism
But set us free from error.
Because yours is the Kingdom and the Power
  and the Song from age to age sealed in faith-
  fulness and truth. Amen.
*(Aramaic Translation of the model prayer
  better known as the "Lord's Prayer")*

3rd STEP:

Three Hail Marys *(said on the set of 3 beads
as we invoke the Light, Love and spiritual
Power of our unfolding soul)*

**Hail Mary, Mother of Earth, the Lords love
Thee. Blessed are You throughout the Universe and blessed are the Children of Humanity.**

Holy Mary, Mother of Gods, nourish us with
wisdom and inspire us through the experience of life and death. Amen.

4th STEP:

One Glory Be *(said on wire before large
single bead)*

**Glory be to the Father-Mother and to the Son
and to the Holy Spirit.**

As it was in the beginning, is now and ever
shall be, world without end. Amen.

O, Lord Jesus, forgive our errors and aid us in our quest.
Lead all souls to Light and Love, especially those most in need of your mercy. Amen.

5th STEP: *(said on large single bead)*

The First Glorious Mystery is known as the Resurrection.
Master Jesus rises from the dead. "He has been raised up; he is not here," so speaks the angel. We are challenged to believe in life after death. We struggle with faith. We remember the chant, "There is no birth, there is no death." Knowing the Soul lives, the Masters beckon us to new understanding and to new realities.

We join together in the saying of the Great Invocation.
From the point of Light within the mind
　of God
Let Light stream forth into the minds of men.
Let Light descend on Earth.

From the point of Love within the Heart
　of God
Let Love stream forth into the hearts of men.
May Christ return to Earth.

From the centre where the Will of God
　is known
Let purpose guide the little wills of men—
The purpose which the Masters know
　and serve.

From the centre which we call the race
  of men
Let the plan of Love and Light work out.
And may it seal the door where evil dwells.

Let Light and Love and Power restore the
  Plan on Earth.

6th STEP:

**Ten Hail Marys as we contemplate, "There
is no death." Life continues to evolve and carries us from form to form as we become increasingly aware of Life itself. We learn to
trust and to know we are each the child of
the Universe and no less than the stars. No
doubt the Universe is unfolding as it should.**

**Hail Mary, Mother of Earth, the Lords love
Thee. Blessed are You throughout the Universe and blessed are the Children of Humanity.**

Holy Mary, Mother of Gods, nourish us with
wisdom and inspire us through the experience of life and death. Amen

7th STEP: *(said on wire before large single bead)*

**Glory be to the Father-Mother and to the Son
and to the Holy Spirit.**

As it was in the beginning, is now and ever
shall be, world without end. Amen.

**O, Lord Jesus, forgive us our errors and aid us
in our quest.**

Lead all souls to Light and Love, especially those most in need of your mercy. Amen.

8th STEP: *(said on large single bead)*

The Second Glorious Mystery is the Ascension.

After speaking, the Lord Jesus ascended into Heaven and took his place in holy service. So too shall our Soul, fulfilled and enlightened, take its place in the world of souls to continue its divine expression in the more subtle planes. The Soul lives and we affirm, "I Am the Soul."

We join together in the saying of the Great Invocation.

From the point of Light within the mind
    of God
Let Light stream forth into the minds of men.
Let Light descend on Earth.

From the point of Love within the Heart
    of God
Let Love stream forth into the hearts of men.
May Christ return to Earth.

From the centre where the Will of God
    is known
Let purpose guide the little wills of men—
The purpose which the Masters know
    and serve.

From the centre which we call the race
    of men
Let the plan of Love and Light work out.

And may it seal the door where evil dwells.

Let Light and Love and Power restore the Plan on Earth.

9th STEP:

Ten Hail Marys as we contemplate the life of the Soul in the higher worlds. We experience brief moments of awareness that help us know the soul nature most often hidden even from ourselves. The Ascension provides the promise, "There is more to life than is revealed. Soul knows life in the subtle worlds."

Hail Mary, Mother of Earth, the Lords love Thee. Blessed are You throughout the Universe and blessed are the Children of Humanity.

Holy Mary, Mother of Gods, nourish us with wisdom and inspire us through the experience of life and death. Amen.

10th STEP: *(said on wire before large single bead)*

Glory be to the Father-Mother and to the Son and to the Holy Spirit.

As it was in the beginning, is now and ever shall be, world without end. Amen.

O, Lord Jesus, forgive us our errors and aid us in our quest.

Lead all souls to Light and Love, especially those most in need of your mercy. Amen.

11th STEP: *(said on large single bead)*

The Third Glorious Mystery is Pentecost.

The outpouring of spiritual gifts fills us with fervor, awareness and the little understood energies of the unfolding spiritual nature. Filled with the Holy Spirit, we will live enlightened lives and bring the energy of the Higher to bless all humanity. According to the gifts that come, we find our way to serve.

We join together in the saying of the Great Invocation.

From the point of Light within the mind
   of God
Let Light stream forth into the minds of men.
Let Light descend on Earth.

From the point of Love within the Heart
   of God
Let Love stream forth into the hearts of men.
May Christ return to Earth.

From the centre where the Will of God
   is known
Let purpose guide the little wills of men—
The purpose which the Masters know
   and serve.

From the centre which we call the race
   of men
Let the plan of Love and Light work out.
And may it seal the door where evil dwells.

Let Light and Love and Power restore the
   Plan on Earth.

12th STEP:

> **Ten Hail Marys as we contemplate the spiritual gifts that unfold as the Lotus of High Consciousness is formed within our nature. Even as the Apostles and Mother Mary received the outpouring, so too shall we experience transmutation and we shall be the chalice into which the Living Fire shall flow.**
>
> **Hail Mary, Mother of Earth, the Lords love Thee. Blessed are You throughout the Universe and blessed are the Children of Humanity.**
>
> Holy Mary, Mother of Gods, nourish us with wisdom and inspire us through the experience of life and death. Amen.

13th STEP: *(said on wire before large single bead)*

> **Glory be to the Father-Mother and to the Son and to the Holy Spirit.**
>
> As it was in the beginning, is now and ever shall be, world without end. Amen.
>
> **O, Lord Jesus, forgive us our errors and aid us in our quest.**
>
> Lead all souls to Light and Love, especially those most in need of your mercy. Amen.

14th STEP: *(said on large single bead)*

> **The Fourth Glorious Mystery is the Assumption.**

The body of the Holy Mother is lifted into
Heaven to continue without decay. The concept of transfiguration of the physical both
mystifies and frightens. Spiritual teachings
tell of Holy Ones who leave no trace of their
physical vehicles, who come and go through
the planes as they serve purposes higher than
our own. We contemplate eternal life with
the Christ, the Masters and the Hierarchy.

**We join together in the saying of the Great
Invocation.**

From the point of Light within the mind
   of God
Let Light stream forth into the minds of men.
Let Light descend on Earth.

From the point of Love within the Heart
   of God
Let Love stream forth into the hearts of men.
May Christ return to Earth.

From the centre where the Will of God
   is known
Let purpose guide the little wills of men—
The purpose which the Masters know
   and serve.

From the centre which we call the race
   of men
Let the plan of Love and Light work out.
And may it seal the door where evil dwells.

Let Light and Love and Power restore the
   Plan on Earth.

15th STEP:

Ten Hail Marys as we contemplate eternal life, the solar initiations, the cosmic initiations and life without end. We seek the grace of an ever unfolding understanding of the Plan of which humanity is a part. The vehicle of Light is being built for all humanity. The pattern has been established. We contemplate new realities as we progress, step by step, into the eternal.

Hail Mary, Mother of Earth, the Lords love Thee. Blessed are You throughout the Universe and blessed are the Children of Humanity.

Holy Mary, Mother of Gods, nourish us with wisdom and inspire us through the experience of life and death. Amen.

16th STEP: *(said on wire before large single bead)*

Glory be to the Father-Mother and to the Son and to the Holy Spirit.

As it was in the beginning, is now and ever shall be, world without end. Amen.

O, Lord Jesus, forgive us our errors and aid us in our quest.

Lead all souls to Light and Love, especially those most in need of your mercy. Amen

17th STEP: *(said on large single bead)*

**The Fifth Glorious Mystery is the Corona-
tion of Mother Mary as Queen of Heaven and
Earth.**

Our attention is focused upon the saints and
sages of all traditions who have guided
humanity to Heaven's door. We come to
know that such as these continue to care for
humanity and to assist us as we go about the
process of becoming Holy Ones ourselves.

**We join together in the saying of the Great
Invocation.**

From the point of Light within the mind
   of God
Let Light stream forth into the minds of men.
Let Light descend on Earth.

From the point of Love within the Heart
   of God
Let Love stream forth into the hearts of men.
May Christ return to Earth.

From the centre where the Will of God
   is known
Let purpose guide the little wills of men—
The purpose which the Masters know
   and serve.

From the centre which we call the race
   of men
Let the plan of Love and Light work out.
And may it seal the door where evil dwells.

Let Light and Love and Power restore the
   Plan on Earth.

18th STEP:

> **Ten Hail Marys as we contemplate the challenges that seek to slow us on our quest. We realize that the difficult steps lead to a great goal. We rededicate ourselves to meeting our challenges well. We take the tests and we love the Holy Ones who have gone before us to show us the sacred way.**
>
> **Hail Mary, Mother of Earth, the Lords love Thee. Blessed are You throughout the Universe and blessed are the Children of Humanity.**
>
> Holy Mary, Mother of Gods, nourish us with wisdom and inspire us through the experience of life and death. Amen

19th STEP: *(said on wire before holy medal)*

> **Glory be to the Father-Mother and to the Son and to the Holy Spirit.**
>
> As it was in the beginning, is now and ever shall be, world without end. Amen.
>
> **O, Lord Jesus, forgive us our errors and aid us in our quest.**
>
> Lead all souls to Light and Love, especially those most in need of your mercy. Amen.

20th STEP: *(said on the holy medal)*

> **Hail, Holy Queen, Mother of Mercy, our Life, our Sweetness and our Hope, to You do we turn our hearts as the awakening Children of**

Eve; to You do we send up our prayers, invoking Your love.

Turn, then, most gracious Advocate, your eyes of mercy toward us, and after this, our period of growth, open to us the kingdom of souls. O clement, O loving, O sweet Mother Mary!

Pray for us, O Holy Mother of Gods, that we may experience the promises of Christ as was willed for us from the beginning. Amen.

This concludes the Glorious Mysteries and ends the third rosary.

Part III

THE MYSTIC ROSARY

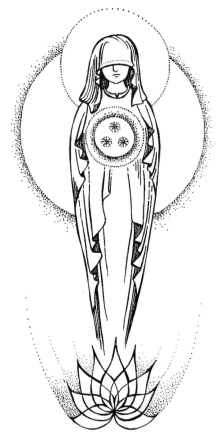

The Veiled Mother of the World

Chapter 8

The Mystic Rosary

PRELUDE TO THE MYSTIC ROSARY

Saint Dominic, from whom the Dominican Order received its name, was born in Spain in 1170. His real name was Domingo de Guzman. As a youth he showed unusual gifts and talents and was educated for the priesthood. His inspirational and persuasive words made him extremely popular, and he was sent on many missionary tours through Spain and France.

In the year 1203 he gathered together a number of young brother Friars to accompany him on his journeys. This marked the beginning of the movement which was to become the Dominican

Chapter reprinted from *The Blessed Virgin Mary, Her Life and Mission,* by Corinne Heline.

97

Order, which attracted some of the most brilliant minds in the Church, many of whom held Chairs in important Colleges throughout Europe. Perhaps the most famous member of the Order was the brilliant Christian philosopher, Thomas Aquinas.

In times of great stress and strain in the outer world, it happens that some of the Great Ones from the inner plane will appear before their chosen messenger to give him strength, courage, inspiration and instruction. And so it was that the Blessed Virgin Mary appeared in a vision to St. Dominic. She gave him the Rosary and taught him much of its magic healing power, which later was demonstrated throughout Spain and France and was afterwards taken into Italy and Ireland.

Many persons today are cognizant of the great spiritual power with which an amulet or an emblem may be invested by means of continuous devotional and reverential usage. This is true of the Cross, which is the principal symbol of Christianity in all Churches. It applies also to the Rose Cross, which is the high symbol of the Rosicrucian Brotherhood. This same truth is applicable to many other emblems, which this limited space does not permit us to enumerate.

The Church is a product of the Piscean Age, which is now drawing to a close. This has been an age of sorrow, pain and tears, and so, appropriately, the principal symbol of the Church is Christ on the Cross.

The New Age Christianity, product of the incoming Aquarian Age, will have for its symbol the liberated and ascended Christ. New Age Christianity teaches that it is possible for man to awaken the innate Christ within himself, and by following the Path of Christian Initiation, which is outlined by the principal Events in the life of Christ Jesus, he may eventually reach the same high place of attainment which is represented by the liberation and ascension of Christ, for each and every man is truly a Christ in the making.

The principal keywords of the Rosary are Adoration, Love and Compassion. Adoration for God, Love for one's fellowman, Compassion for the sufferings of all living creatures on the earth planet.

The Rosary possesses a rich heritage of mystic or hidden meanings. It is some of these inner truths which we have endeavored to touch upon in this chapter. Therefore, it is titled The Chapter of the Mystic Rosary.

The serious aspirant comes to realize the magic powers of meditation. He learns that it is possible to take a passage of Scripture or a few lines from a poem, and through continuous meditation and prayer it will become a mantra of power. Such was the use of King David's Psalms, and it was for this purpose that they were written and used in the Temples of his day.

The early Christian used the Psalms in the same way, and often they were divided into three parts, each containing fifty Psalms. Early hermit monks describe these three designations by knotted ropes which they wore tied around their waist.

In the third volume of the New Age Bible Interpretations we have endeavored to show the various purposes of the Psalms. Some are mantras for physical healing, others for mental renewal and still others are to be used for purity and transmutation, while many hold keys to definite forms of Initiation.

When a certain number of prayers came to be ascribed to the Blessed Mary they were termed Our Lady's Psalm. Later it was natural that the name Rosary was chosen to describe them, for the rose had been a key to the varied forms of Initiation since the beginning of time when the first Mysteries were given to mankind.

THE MYSTIC ROSARY

The Mysteries of the Rosary outline the most important Steps in the Path of the Christian Mystics, illustrated in the lives of the two greatest Beings who ever came to live upon this plane, namely, the blessed Lord Christ Jesus and the beloved Mary of Bethlehem.

The Mysteries of the Rosary in the life of the Lord Christ began with the Nativity and ended with the Ascension.

The Mysteries of the Rosary in the life of the beautiful Mary began with the Annunciation and ended with the Assumption and the Crowning by the Christ in Heaven.

These high events in the lives of these two illustrious Beings give the perfect type-pattern of the Christed Man and the Perfect Woman and have been exemplified on earth for the emulation of all mankind.

The early Christian Fathers, notably Origen and St. Augustine, made frequent allusions to the Mysteries upon which the early Christian Church was founded. St. Augustine stated specifically that there was a hidden wisdom for the Few and outer teaching for the majority. When the Church discarded initiation, this inner wisdom was largely forgotten; however, certain ceremonials and rituals which formed the outer covering for these high truths continued to exist, but the key to their real meaning had been entirely lost.

The most fascinating phase of the work for the mystic Christian is the rediscovery of this long forgotten wisdom. It is for this reason that we have entitled this study The Mystic Rosary. We are not concerned with the teaching of the Church concerning the Rosary; we are interested only in discovering something of the vast wealth of its inner meaning.

Pythagoras states that all creation is centered in Number—and the numerological symbology of

the Rosary will prove to be one of the most fascinating phases of its study. We note that the Rosary is divided into five equal parts, each part
containing ten beads. There are four large beads
which separate these five parts. Ten is the number of man and woman walking hand in hand up
the Path of Illumination. One has always been a
symbol of deity, or divinity. It typifies God in the
heavens and the God-power or consciousness of
All-Good which is latent in every human being.
The chief purpose of attainment is to awaken
and bring into manifestation the latent divinity
within humanity.

Ten and One is eleven, which is a number of
magical power. It symbolizes the development
of Balance or Equilibrium within man and is
known esoterically as Polarity, which is the
highest attainment of the Initiatory Path and
was known among the early Christians as the
Rite of the Mystic Marriage.

The four large beads also represent the most
priceless gifts the Lord Christ brought to
mankind. Excepting for the very Few, such as the
Disciples on the Day of Pentecost, the priceless
Truths are entirely unheeded and unknown—al-
though they should form a component part of
the Christian religion. They cannot be given to
man until he proves himself worthy to receive
them, which he has not yet done. We only talk
about Christ's teachings, but we do not live
them. Just so long as we, both as nations and individuals, are content to follow the Old Dispen-

sation law of, "An eye for an eye and a tooth for a tooth" instead of having exchanged this for the precepts of the Golden Rule, "Do unto others as you would have them do unto you," we are not truly living up to the high precepts of the Christ teaching. And so down through the ages it has been but the Few who have been worthy to follow the footsteps of the Immortal Twelve and have bestowed upon them the powers which the First Disciples received on the Day of Pentecost, known as the First of the Great Christ Mysteries.

The pendulum of the Rosary to which the Crucifix is attached consists of three beads guarded on each side by a larger bead—which gives us also the numbers Three and Five.

The Mysteries of the Rosary are also divided into three parts, and each mystery consists of five steps. Hence we note that three and five are both important numbers to be considered in numbers, denoting perfection and as such occupies an important place in all world religions.

Three is the number of the Holy Trinity—one of the highest tenets of the Christian faith. Three is formed of One (masculine) and Two (feminine), and from this union is born the number Three, whether it occurs upon the physical, mental or spiritual plane. For example, it is the God Power, or Will principle, which unites with the Christ or Wisdom Principle, and from this union is born the Third or Activity Principle which is known as the Power of the Holy Ghost.

As we meditate upon this Truth we can better comprehend the meaning of Pythagoras' words, "All creation is counted in Number."

Five is formed through the union of the odd or masculine number Three and the feminine number Two. While this number implies union, it does not necessarily imply harmony. Five is a number of Life and is ever seeking and searching for something higher than it knows, so Five is considered the Number of the Great Quest. Thus we may see the importance of the Three and Five in the symbolic study of the Rosary. Three typifies Perfection or Attainment, and Five the quest or search which leads finally to that attainment.

The life of the aspirant in the old Piscean Age, which is now closing, was vastly different from that of the aspirant of the new Aquarian Age now dawning. The aspirant of the old age was largely a recluse shutting himself away from the world and spending his time in study, meditation and various forms of self-mortification. The keynotes of the New Age are Unity and Brotherhood. The aspirant lives his life in the outer, busy world dedicating himself in loving self-forgetting service for the betterment of all whom he contacts. His pursuits are all dedicated to furthering the ideals of Universal Brotherhood and World Unity.

The Lord Christ is the perfect type-pattern for the aspirant's emulation—the supreme ideal being that the Christ may be born in him. Consequently he, too, passes through many similar events to those outlined in the life of the Christ.

The three Mysteries of the Rosary are divided into the Joyous, the Sorrowful and the Glorious. These typify the various life experiences which the aspirant meets in his daily living for after all, life is the supreme Initiator and formed of both sadness and joy, of tears and laughter, or sickness and health, of shadow and sunshine and of life and death.

The Sorrowful Mysteries

It is a well-known fact that we gain more through sorrow than through joy. The Christ made this plain when He said, "If ye would be my disciples ye must take up your cross and follow Me"--there is no other way. One of the tenets of the orthodox church today is that you must learn to bear the cross before you will be found worthy to wear the crown. We have quoted so often that beautiful statement taken from "Light on the Path," which is so brief, and which every aspirant who has entered the Path knows to be so true—"Before the feet can stand in the presence of the Masters they must be washed in the blood of the heart."

The more advanced the ego, the more severe will be the testings which are given to him. This is the meaning of the biblical statement, "Whom God loveth He chasteneth." One of the most severe tests which an aspirant can ever know is the loss of the best-loved. Sometimes this occurs through death and, again, as an even more severe test, a voluntary renunciation for the sake of a greater good for others. One who passes this way knows well the meaning of the Crucifixion. The Blessed Virgin passed through this agony during the long hours when she stood at the foot of the Cross. Another severe testing is that the ego, compelled by the force of destiny, may be born amid uncongenial surroundings and be reared in completely incompatible companionship. The force of circumstances may cause this bondage to endure for many years— sometimes for an entire life. Such a one learns to know well the Agony of the Garden.

Another severe testing is that in which one may live for many years in the closest relationship with a long-trusted friend or in a marital relationship of peace and harmony—suddenly to discover that the companion or friend so trusted and beloved, had proven to be entirely unworthy of that love and confidence. To such a one the Way of the Cross becomes an all too familiar way.

Another severe testing may come when after years of work and personal sacrifice a promising career in some loved work has been successfully achieved, when suddenly without warning, by means of disease or accident, the physical body becomes incapacitated and one is compelled to live on with only the sorrowful memories of what might have been.

To such a one the pain of the Scourging becomes all too familiar and he knows too well the weight of the Crown of Thorns.

The Joyful Mysteries

As we have frequently stated, the Blessed Virgin Mary belongs to no one church or creed, race or nation. Her work and her message are world-wide and are primarily for the upliftment and betterment of all womankind. She will continue to work close to the earth plane until woman's equality shall have been attained socially, economically, politically, educationally and spiritually.

As previously stated, the Christ is the perfect type-pattern for the emulation of all mankind, and the Events of His Life find their prototype in the various experiences which the aspirant meets upon the Path. The same is true in relation to the life of the Blessed Virgin Mary. She came to earth as the perfect type-pattern of womanhood—and as motherhood is the brightest jewel in a woman's crown, the Blessed Virgin also expresses the supreme ideal of perfect motherhood.

In the incoming New Age the Annunciation will become an actual experience in the lives of the most advanced women of the New Race. In the humanity of that day conception will be angel guided and angel directed. Aquarius is the home of the angelic Hierarchy and their varied, beautiful and important ministry for this earth planet will become better understood and appreciated. There are hosts of ministering Angels who guide and direct every phase of evolution upon this earth. There are bands of Nature Angels who direct the growth of plants and flowers. There are other Angels who work with every form of animal life and still others who work with every form of human life from the most primitive to the most advanced.

There are some Few upon the earth who are conscious of the closeness of these angelic guardians; however, the vast majority remain totally unaware of their close proximity, and many are skeptical of their very existence.

In the New Age now dawning the most advanced women will be chosen to become the mothers of the great Masters and Teachers who will come to inspire and illumine the entire race. These advanced women will be placed in schools during that most sacred and important interval in a woman's life, namely the prenatal epoch. Their environment will consist only of those things which are high, noble and true. They will hear only the greatest music, meditate upon the high works of art, read books expressive of the noblest sentiments and think thoughts of purity and truth. In other words they will be taught in all ways to emulate the perfect pattern given to womankind by the Blessed Virgin Mary.

One of the most beautiful events recorded in the Bible is known as The Visitation. It was during this most sacred time of the prenatal epoch that the Blessed Virgin spent several months in the home of her cousin, Elizabeth, who was also an expectant mother, and it was here that these two Initiate women were in conscious communication with the two great Master Egos who were to take Earth embodiment through them, namely the Holy Master Jesus and John the Baptist, of whom Christ Jesus said there was never one born upon the earth greater than he. This same beautiful ideal will also be consummated by women of the New Age as they are being prepared for their sublime ministry of perfected motherhood. At this time each birth will become a Holy Nativity. Every incoming ego, surrounded by hosts of chorusing Angels, will descend, enfolded in vast waves of glorious Light, to enter painlessly and beautifully into the heart of the expectant and happy Mother. The Presentation in the Temple will become a time of high dedication for both the mother and the child. This presentation will not be under the auspices of churchly priests but under the direction of guardian Angels. It is here that in the Akashic Records, or Memory of Nature both mother and child will be taught to study their own earth destiny and the mission which they have come into physical embodiment to fulfill. Under angelic direction they will be shown the high lights, or decisive events of their earth mission and will be instructed how best to use their own free will and wise discrimination in bringing these Events to their highest and noblest fulfillment.

The Fifth Step in the Joyous Mysteries is the finding of the Christ Child in the Temple. We are all familiar with the biblical story of the sorrow of Mary and Joseph when the Christ Child was lost for three days during their journey from Jerusalem, and their great joy upon finding Him discoursing with the Teachers in the Temple. This Event also has its prototype in the life of the aspirant. The temple represents the human body which the disciple is taught to purify and perfect so it becomes truly a fit dwelling place for the Christ Light latent within man himself. As the aspirant advances along the Path, this Christ Light increasingly awakens within himself and becomes the wise teacher guiding and directing the awakened ego at all times and in all circumstances.

It is here that the Path is extremely narrow and surrounded on all sides by many pitfalls. If one does not live always to the highest that he knows, it is very easy to lose contact with this inner Light which illumines and nourishes the higher nature.

The Psalms are Hymns of Initiation. Many of these Psalms are Songs of Sorrow because of certain mistakes or misdeeds by which this inner contact has been broken. Others are Songs of great Rejoicing, when by means of repentance, reform and sometimes restitution, this contact with the divine Light within has been re-established.

Again we reiterate the Life itself is the Supreme Initiator, and it depends on how well we learn to meet these experiences, which are enumerated both as the Sorrowful and the Joyful Mysteries, and to extract the essence of these experiences, converting them into additional soul Light, soul Life and soul Power, that we shall be able to demonstrate our readiness and our worthiness to take part in these glorious Mysteries.

The Glorious Mysteries

The Rite of the Resurrection in the life of the disciple marks the ability to function consciously apart from the physical body both in the inner and outer planes. We are all familiar with the beautiful Rosicrucian prayer, "While my body is peacefully resting in sleep may I still be found faithfully working in the vineyard of Christ, for as spirit I need no rest."

The disciple is taught first to function consciously apart from the physical body during the hours of sleep, and still later, in more advanced teaching he is taught first to be able to leave the body at will during the hours of either day or night in response to calls for help that may come either from the earth plane or invisible realms.

There is nothing fantastic or unrealistic about such teaching, as it has always been familiar to the esoteric Christian. As an example of this we quote St. Paul as he refers to his initiatory experience in II Cor: Ch 12, V3-4, "I knew a man in Christ about fourteen years ago (whether in the body, I cannot tell; or whether out of the body, I cannot tell: God knoweth), such a one caught up to the third heaven. And I knew such a man (whether in the body or out of the body, I cannot tell: God knoweth), how that he was caught up into paradise and heard unspeakable things which it is not lawful for a man to utter."

It is impossible in so limited a space to even begin to describe the wonderful revelations of the inner planes; here the student will find great libraries far beyond his highest dreams. The artist will revel in colors of which earth-dulled physical eyes can have no concept. The musician will take joy in the celestial music of angelic choirs. Whatever one's life interest has been here upon earth, there he will find it in its perfected form. Perhaps one of the most wonderful experiences of being permitted to function consciously in the higher realms is the ability to know from first-hand personal knowledge *that there is no death*— and that all life is continuous and eternal. After such exalted experiences, one returns to earth to join with St. Paul in his exultant chant, "O death where is thy sting? O grave, where is thy victory?"

The Rite of the Ascension in the life of the disciple represents the ability to ascend into ever higher and wider realms for the purpose of added service and the gaining of higher wisdom. The wonders and the glories of these higher realms can never be adequately described in human language. We can only say that Infinity is the keyword of these higher spheres and "Onward and Upward Forever" is the mantra given to the disciple as he continues in this glorious Way.

Orthodox Christianity teaches that one must die before he can know the glories of the heaven worlds. Esoteric Christianity teaches that it is possible by means of Initiation, learning to function consciously apart from the physical body, to know the wonders and the glories of these high realms here and now, while we are still living upon the earth.

As has been previously stated, the descent of the Holy Ghost upon the disciples on that great Day of Pentecost was a part of the teaching given to the Immortal Twelve when they were initiated into the First of the Great Christ Mysteries. This is the destined attainment awaiting the entire human race at the end of the present Earth Period.

We noted in the Joyous Mysteries, the Presentation in the Temple, that both the Mother and the Child will be dedicated and consecrated for their high earth mission. In this, the Third of the Glorious Mysteries, the disciple is dedicated and consecrated both for his work upon the earth plane and also for his mission in the higher spiritual realms.

At the time of the Assumption of the Blessed Virgin Mary she was the perfect type pattern for all humankind when the race is ready to receive the Second of the Great Christ Mysteries. She had learned the conquest of all physical substance, hence the physical earth and the physical body held no more lessons for her, and therefore she was freed from both. In the Assumption the Blessed Virgin passed into the Etheric Realms, there to make her home among the Angels. The lowest body in which Angels function is formed of etheric substance. They can, therefore, only be seen on earth by those having etheric sight or extended vision. This is why the many beautiful and important Angelic ministries for the earth are unseen and uncomprehended by the vast majority of persons on earth.

The Blessed Virgin Mary, however, voluntarily sacrifices much of her time in those realms of bliss and remains close to the earth to work for the upliftment of the human race and will continue to do so until her high mission has been fulfilled.

The highest attainment that anyone on this earth plane can ever know is to be found worthy to be lifted up into the presence of the Blessed Lord Christ and to receive His blessing. To listen to that wondrous Voice with its loving intonations as He says, "Well done, thou good and faithful servant—enter thou into the joy of thy Lord."

This was the supreme attainment of the Blessed Virgin Mary when, at the time of the Assumption, she was crowned by our Lord Christ as the Queen of Angels and Men.

"Now, let woman—the Mother of the World—
say, 'Let there be Light,' and let her affirm her
fiery achievements. What will this Light be like,
and which of her achievements will be the great
fiery ones? The banner of spirit will be raised,
and upon it will be inscribed 'Love, Knowledge
and Beauty.' Yes, only the heart of the woman,
the mother, may gather under this Banner the
children of the whole world, without distinc-
tions of sex, race, nationality and religion."

Helena Roerich
October 7, 1930

APPENDIX

MAKING YOUR OWN ROSARY

Centuries ago, when knighthood was in flower, a popular way to make rosary beads was to use fragrant rose petals and cook them down to make a dough. This dough-like substance could then be rolled into small beads and strung by making a hole through each bead. The delicate scent of roses was released when the beads were warmed by wearing and lingered for some time. The rose has been known as the flower of Our Lady, so these beads were particularly treasured.

In recent years this once popular method of making rose beads has been rediscovered. Information about this process may be obtained by contacting:

Rosebeades
Box 1994
Fayetteville, AR   72702

GLOSSARY

AKASHIC RECORDS. The mental and emotional imprint of an individual or group memory held in the astral body.

"ALL IS READY, MASTER. COME." A special chant used at Wesak celebration but most significant as one stands ready to receive great outpourings of grace.

AQUARIAN AGE. A cycle of time wherein Earth receives the influence of the constellation Aquarius in a specific way, astronomically and astrologically.

ARCHETYPE. A pattern or blueprint held in the inner planes to guide and assist the lower planes in forming or evolving.

ASPIRANT. One who is consciously walking the spiritual path of initiation.

ASPIRATION. The stimulation of high ideals or images for the benefit of devotion; use of deity to uplift human values.

ASTRAL SENSES. Senses which psychically perceive the less dense or more subtle frequencies, i.e., feelings or thoughts.

ASTRAL VEHICLE. The astral body, less material than the physical body, is the emotional matter interpenetrating the physical body.

119

AVALOKITA. Sanskrit for "the Lord who is perceived or cognized"; the spiritual entity whose influence is perceived and felt; the Soul unfolded and expressing, as in adept or Master.

AWAKENED ONES. Those aware of deity and in action with higher realities.

BASIC SELF (OR BASIC NATURE). The personality we choose—like a tool box—to come into this life, possessing certain characteristics such as masculine and feminine traits; more than what is usually meant by the term subconscious.

BODHISATTVA. Sanskrit for one who carries the Buddhic energy and in a future incarnation will become a Buddha (enlightened to Nirvana); used much as Western spirituality uses "Christed."

CATHOLIC. Latin for universal, all-inclusive.

CHAKRA CENTERS. Actual vortices of force existing in the etheric bodies of human beings, which correspond to different levels of consciousness, and control the physical condition of the area of the body which they influence.

CHALICE. The receptive mind; the open high consciousness that can receive inspiration, vision and straight knowledge from the Christ; the receiver of energies from Spiritual Triad.

CHANTING. Repetitive vocalizing—spoken or sung—designed to penetrate the subconscious to affect the life of an aspirant.

CHRIST-WITHIN. The divine nature within a human soul; a spark or seed of the Divine with the potential of being fostered into a conscious awareness attuned to the Christ, Masters and teachers of angels and humans; living in the Christ Presence.

CHRISTED MAN. The evolved human in whom "the mind that is in Christ Jesus be also in you" is made manifest.

CHRISTIAN INITIATION. A process within esoteric Christianity describing stages of growth; five major steps are called birth, baptism, transfiguration, crucifixion-resurrection, ascension.

CLOUD OF KNOWABLE THINGS. The vast awareness into which flows the mind of God.

COLLECTIVE UNCONSCIOUS. Sum total of all levels of mind existing below the threshold of conscious awareness for all of humanity.

CONSCIOUSNESS. The spark of divinity in the human; the ensouling energy that is the root of all awareness.

CONTEMPLATION. Similar to meditation; the act of holding a thought or object before the mental vision and observing the thought from many perspectives.

COSMIC HEART. The "spiritual heart" of the universe.

DECADE. A pattern (set) of ten repetitive prayers used in saying rosaries.

DENSE BODY. The physical body.

DESCENT INTO MATTER. The soul enveloped into denser and denser realities culminating in a physical or materialized result.

DEVOTION. Emotion generated in the astral body uplifted and directed toward a high ideal of Goodness, Truth and Love, sometimes toward a deity or individual.

DHARMA LIGHT. An Eastern term for the outpouring of love, mind and will of God; Dharma is that which comes as the grace of God poured out upon the earth, sometimes shortened to "good karma."

DISCIPLE. A third degree initiate.

DIVINE FEMININE. The feminine aspect of God; the perfection of the female principle; divine love; the nurturing Mother aspect of God.

DIVINE REALIZATION. The synthesizing of revelation or awareness in relationship to soul or higher awareness, the moments of inspiration coming together into a whole.

ENLIGHTENMENT. Supreme discrimination; a state of mind filled with spiritual wisdom.

ERA OF WOMAN. Esoteric teachings offer the ideas of the Age of Aquarius as a balancing of the nature (masculine-feminine) of humanity through an awakening to the values of the feminine influence.

ESOTERIC. An inner or out-of-sight process; hidden or secret teachings given only to those who are spiritually ready to receive them.

ESOTERIC CHRISTIANITY. The Christian tradition contains an esoteric and an exoteric level of understanding. The esoteric focuses upon the developing of the Christ-Within and the gifts of the spirit, as referred to in the New Testament; esoteric Christianity is equivalent to mystical Christianity. The exoteric Christian tradition focuses upon dogma and rites and forms the better understood practices of the church and church tradition.

ESOTERICISM. Teachings emphasizing keys to the inner nature or soul development.

ETHERIC. Having to do with the frequencies interpenetrating and beyond the earth's atmosphere; a subtle matter less dense than physical from which springs everything in the physical world.

EVOCATION. The coming forth of energy in response to an invocation.

EXOTERIC. Outer, public religious practices that are not confined to an inner circle of disciples or initiates; teachings to which the keys have not been openly given; the opposite of esoteric or hidden.

FEMININE PRINCIPLE. The feminine aspect of God often called the Mother, especially concerned with love, sensitivity and nurturing; usually associated with intuition and help.

GOD IMMINENT. The God within creation.

GOD TRANSCENDENT. The God of human affairs above and beyond the world.

GREAT COSMIC MOTHER. The space that receives creation and gives birth, nurtures and sustains life.

GREAT WHOLENESS. A recognition of the Creator; a title for "About Whom Naught Can Be Said."

GURU. Sanskrit for teacher; one who brings light (awareness) to the spiritual and intellectual parts (soul) of the disciple; spiritual teacher; a master in metaphysical and ethical doctrines; one who represents and reflects high consciousness to and for the disciple.

HIERARCHY. The delegated, directive supreme authority and power overseeing planetary life on the higher planes which directs, guides and teaches initiates and disciples; also known as the Great White Brotherhood or orders/brotherhoods of initiated souls working as a field of intelligence serving the Father.

HUMAN GROUP MIND. The collective consciousness/unconsciousness of humanity, as per Carl Jung; humanity's joint akashic record, as per Eastern symbology.

ILLUSION. The imperfect recognition of reality as truth; a false interpretation; a mirage. In occultism everything finite (like the universe and all in it) is called illusion or maya.

INITIATION. A process of awakening to one's true identity and using it in the service of humanity; the practice of admission into sacred teachings or organizations; entrance into the spiritual life; process of understanding or expansion of consciousness.

INTUITION. Spiritual perception; a wisdom of the heart; divine knowing, often called the sixth sense; a direct way of sensing subtle influences. This sense is designed to aid one to know divine love, thought and will.

INVOCATION. To call forth energy.

ISIS. Egyptian diety; personification of Divine Mother.

JESUS CHRIST. The initiate Jesus served Christ, head of Hierarchy, by building purified lower vehicles of high frequency for His use. Jesus became one with the planetary Christ.

KABALIST. One who studies and practices the Hebrew mystery teachings, the Kabalah, and interprets the hidden meaning of the Scriptures.

KAMA-MANAS. Sanskrit for lower or reincarnating ego; the lower mind or animal soul.

KUAN YIN. The Eastern name given to the feminine deity which appears from time to time to inspire and comfort humanity, known as the Bodhisattva of Compassion.

LIGHT. A degree of electrical energy which, when condensed, forms matter; a visible proxy on earth of the invisible Deity; often used as a symbol of mind or thought, especially in regard to divine mind.

LORD MAITREYA. A name used by Eastern spiritual paths as the guiding consciousness that would permeate humanity with an awakening of the God-Within; used by esotericists as an Eastern word for the Christ.

MALA. A set of prayer beads used in the Eastern tradition to invoke spiritual power.

MANTRA. A program of incantations spoken to the subconscious, sometimes aloud, sometimes silently, used to reprogram and to train one for new awareness.

MANTRA YOGA. A particular practice using affirmations, chants, words and prayers to increase the connection to God and to experience the Holy Presence. Mantra Yoga is considered a seventh ray approach.

MARIAN YEAR. The year dedicated to Mary for her intercession on behalf of humanity; i.e., 1987 was declared by Pope John Paul as the Marian Year for Peace.

MASCULINE PRINCIPLE. The masculine aspect of God
usually called the Father; especially concerned
with will, intellect or law.

MASTER. One who has his higher principles
awakened and lives them; one who develops an individual consciousness or recognition of his oneness with God; a fifth degree initiate; one who
achieves "self-mastery" in spiritual matters.

MEDITATION. Techniques vary; however, the goal is
to listen inwardly and to be receptive to inner
knowing.

MENTAL NATURE. The mental body, the mental plane
is that part or aspect of nature which belongs to
consciousness working as a plane thought, being
organized into various functions or levels of mind.

MENTAL VEHICLE. Name given to the organized parts
of mental planes wherein one is centered and able
to utilize consciousness.

MOTHER PRINCIPLE. The feminine principle in creation; the Mother aspect of the Deity; that receptive part that accepts the spirit aspect in order to
manifest in matter.

MYSTERIES, THE. Each series of the rosary focuses
upon the life of Jesus, the Christ, in a particular
way: the Joyous Mysteries focus upon Jesus preparing his will to serve the Christ; the Sorrowful
focus upon the path of the initiate and the
Glorious offer humanity glimpses of the unknown
world of spirit. The contemplation of a life so
divine is for the purpose of penetrating into a
greater purpose in life than that easily seen from
the personality level.

MYSTERIES OF ISIS. Secret teachings of Ancient Egypt regarding the Mother of Osiris and the deity referred to as Mother of Humanity (pre-Christian).

MYSTIC CHRISTIAN. One who seeks to know oneness with the Christ through experience rather than mind.

NEW ADAM. Born of a divine idea through the overshadowing of the Holy Spirit. Often this title is used to denote the emerging, new, more-aware human on the path of evolution back to the source.

NEW AGE. A shift in consciousness that occurs within individuals as they leave behind the old view that has served them and must begin to build a new perspective appropriate to the breakthrough in consciousness they have experienced. Using New Age as a point in time is popular currently as it occurs for the masses at the same time as the Age of Aquarius dawns. Example: Master Jesus was New Age when he presented his disciples with a new vision, i.e., the good news of his ministry.

NEW JERUSALEM. A prototype city in heaven that is the home of spiritual beings; usually thought of as Shamballa in Eastern teachings.

OMNIPOTENCE. All-powerful; having unlimited or universal power, authority or force.

PATH OF INITIATION. The spiritual evolution of souls; the process of becoming enlightened through dedicated self-mastery and descriptive steps useful to help one determine work to be done upon self.

PHYLACTERY. Two small leather boxes containing strips of parchment inscribed with quotations from the Hebrew scriptures which are used by Jewish men during morning worship; it invokes physical action, repetitive prayer and the holding of thoughts in contemplation/meditation.

PISCEAN Age. A cycle of time wherein the Earth received the influence of the constellation Pisces in a specific way according to astronomy and astrology; roughly calculated as from about the time of Master Jesus' birth until 1987.

PLAN, THE. The Higher Plan or design for one's life or for the life of the planet.

PLANETARY CHRIST. The Christ, head of Hierarchy, who reigns supreme over the planet and its hierarchy, angels and men; the guiding consciousness of the planet.

RAYS. Seven energy or vibrational expressions of God; qualities of the divine nature.

RELIGION. A system of dogma and creeds used to guide the outer life in expression of belief in a supernatural power. Religion forms a specific pattern or dogma—the way experienced, given, received and lived by prophets or inspired ones and used by others to aid in spiritual growth.

RISEN CHRIST. The Christ of Easter morning who demonstrated mastery over death.

SEED THOUGHT. Phrase designed to put one in a posture to penetrate the veil separating rational mind and inspired mind. Thinking upon these phrases, our mind penetrates the veiled, rational meaning and begins to perceive the "more meaningful" thought. Seed thoughts are dehydrated thought; meditating upon them is designed to reconstitute the greater meaning.

SHAKTI. Sanskrit for the Supreme or Divine Mother; the energies or active powers of the deities represented as awakening or unfolding influences or energies; the feminine aspect of a god power.

SPIRITUAL. Having to do with the evolving of the inner soul; spirit is Latin for breath, ritual is Latin for rites—the combination, spirit-ritual, meaning breath-rites.

STRAIGHT KNOWLEDGE. Revelation; knowledge received from the consciousness of the presence of God.

SUBCONSCIOUS. The storehouse of knowledge held individually or collectively in the mind to be utilized by various levels of mind, consciously or not.

SUPERCONSCIOUS. High self; God self.

TARA. Revered by Mongols and Tibetans as a female emanation of Avalokita, a female Master.

TRANSCENDENTAL. Surpassing the senses; mystical.

TRANSPERSONAL. Transcending or reaching beyond the personal or individual nature.

VEHICLE. Occult word for body.

VEIL. A protective covering used to secret the perception mechanism of the expanding mind. Veils dissolve as consciousness heightens and perception clears.

WAYSHOWER. A prophet or enlightened one who has gone before humanity to lead the Way; each Wayshower lays out a system to aid others in finding their own expression.

WISDOM TEACHINGS. A collection of wisdom or body of knowledge on the hidden nature of humanity and the world held sacred through all time; the purpose of studying it is for the attainment of wisdom and awakening the spiritual memory of the soul.

WORRY STONE. Small, pebble-like stones used in the Huna system for invoking spiritual power, especially employed in rites of healing or the saying of affirmations.

YOGA. Practices designed to help bring about union of spirit and matter (soul and personality).

"YOU ARE GODS." We are reminded in the Old and New Testaments that we are Gods; the feminine principle of life is to bring this about.

INDEX

A

Active Intelligence, 29, 31, 103
  and The Glorious Mysteries, 41,
    79
  and the mysteries, 41
Adam, new, 13
Age
  of enlightenment, 27
  of Patriarchs, 19
  Piscean, 32, 46, 98, 104
  ray influence of, 30
  See also Middle Ages
Agony of the Garden, 106
  See also Sorrowful Mysteries,
    first
Akashic Records, 109
Ancient Wisdom, 33
Annunciation, 101
  and the New Age, 107
  See Joyful Mysteries, first
Aquarian Age
  and Divine Mother, 20
  as accompanies New Age, 127
  as Era of Woman, 26, 122
  change from Piscean, 32, 104
  Christianity in, 99
  cross of Risen Christ in, 46
  mystery tradition in, 42
  mystic way of, 42
  seventh ray influence of, 32
The Aquarian Gospel of Jesus
  the Christ, 7
Aquarian Waterbearer, *Illus.*, xix
Aquinas, Thomas, 98
Asanas, 6
Ascension, 100, 112, 121
  See also Glorious Mysteries,
    second
Aspirant, 11, 14, 99
  and courage, 71

  as world server, 42
  awakening of Christ Light in, 110
  in Aquarian Age, 104
  in Eastern tradition, 6
  in the past, 104
  life experiences of, 105
  severe tests, 105
  task of, 40
Aspiration, 16, 30
Aspirations, 10
Assumption, 101, 113 – 114
  See also Glorious Mysteries,
    fourth
Astara School, 23
Astral body, 7, 10
Augustine, Saint, 101
Aura, 11, 24
Autobiography of a Yogi, 22
Avalokita, 36
Avatar, 34
  See also Lord Maitreya

B

Babaji, 22 – 23
Baptism, 121
Basic self, 4
Beads, 4, 17, 42
  complete set, 48
  decades of, 39 – 40, 102
  from rose petals, 117
  large, in Rosary, 102
  See also Rosary
Birth, 121
Blavatsky, H. P., 11
Blofeld, John, 36
Bodhisattva of Compassion
  See Kuan Yin
Brain
  arcing of hemispheres, 15 – 16
  left hemisphere, 15 – 16
  masculine hemisphere, 15

Do you need additional copies of *The Aquarian Rosary* for friends or a group?

We encourage you to support your local bookstore. But if they are out of stock, simply use this handy order form.

❏ Please send _____ copies of *The Aquarian Rosary* at $9.95 plus $1.50 shipping. My check or money order is enclosed.

❏ Please send a catalog of other books and teaching tapes.

Name_____

Address_____

City_____

State_____Zip_____

Send order & payment to

Village Book Store

22 Summit Ridge Dr. • Tahlequah, OK 74465
(918) 456-3421

Do you need additional copies of *The Aquarian Rosary* for friends or a group?

We encourage you to support your local bookstore. But if they are out of stock, simply use this handy order form.

❏   Please send _____copies of *The Aquarian Rosary* at $9.95 plus $1.50 shipping. My check or money order is enclosed.

❏   Please send a catalog of other books and teaching tapes.

Name_____

Address_____

City_____

State_____Zip_____

Send order & payment to
Village Book Store
22 Summit Ridge Dr. • Tahlequah, OK 74465
(918) 456-3421

Rosaries and Risen-Christ crosses available in various styles and prices. For information on current stock, call or write:
Village Gift Shop
22 Summit Ridge Dr.•Tahlequah, OK 74464
(800) 386-7161 or (918) 456-3421